The Technical, Scientific and Medical Publishing Market

by Judith S. Duke

Knowledge Industry Publications, Inc.
White Plains, NY and London

Communications Library

The Technical, Scientific and Medical Publishing Market

Library of Congress Cataloging in Publication Data

Duke, Judith S.
  The technical, scientific, and medical publishing market.

  (Communications library)
  Includes index.
  1. Technical publishing. 2. Science publishing.
3. Medical publishing. 4. Market surveys. I. Title.
II. Series.
Z286.T4D84 1985   070.5   84-26163
ISBN 0-86729-084-6

Printed in the United States of America

Copyright © 1985 by Knowledge Industry Publications, Inc., 701 Westchester Ave., White Plains, NY 10604. Not to be reproduced in any form whatever without written permission from the publisher.

10   9   8   7   6   5   4   3   2   1

Table of Contents

List of Tables iv

1 Introduction 1
2 Size and Structure of the TSM Information Market 7
3 Books 25
4 Magazines and Journals... 67
5 Newsletters and Loose-Leaf Services............................ 107
6 Database Publishing: Print and Online 131
7 Conclusions... 167
8 Profiles of Major TSM Publishers 173

Index.. 210

About the Author 217

List of Tables

Table 2.1:	Estimated Size of the Market for Technical, Scientific and Medical Books Information, 1975 and 1982	8
Table 2.2:	Scientists by Field of Specialization, and Engineers, 1976 and 1980	9
Table 2.3:	College Enrollment in Science and Engineering Curricula, 1972, 1974 and 1980	10
Table 2.4:	Earned Degrees Conferred in the Sciences, 1972 and 1979-1980	11
Table 2.5:	Number of Physicians, Dentists and Nurses in the U.S. and Schools for Same, Selected Years, 1950 to 1980	12
Table 2.6:	Physicians by Specialty, 1970, 1975 and 1980	13
Table 2.7:	U.S. Physicians and Dentists, by State, 1980	14
Table 2.8:	Persons Employed in Selected Health Occupations, 1975 and 1981	16
Table 2.9:	Outlays for Scientific Research and Development, 1972-1982	16
Table 2.10:	Total National Health Expenditures on Medical Research, 1970 and 1975-1982	17
Table 3.1:	Sales of Professional Books, Technical and Scientific Books, Medical Books and Total Book Industry Sales, 1972-1982	28
Table 3.2:	Index of Technical and Scientific Book Sales, Medical Book Sales and Total Industry Sales Compared with Gross National Product, 1972-1982	30
Table 3.3:	Trends in Technical, Scientific and Medical Book Titles, 1970-1982	31
Table 3.4	Estimated Revenue of Six Leading Scientific and Technical Book Publishers, 1980	34
Table 3.5:	Estimated Revenue of Eight Leading Medical Book Publishers, 1980	37
Table 3.6:	Sales of Technical and Scientific Books and Medical Books, by Type of Customer, 1982	41
Table 3.7:	U.S. Exports of Technical, Scientific and Professional Books and Total U.S. Book Exports, 1977-1982	50
Table 3.8:	Net Sales of Technical, Scientific and Medical Books, by Geographic Location, 1982	51
Table 3.9:	Operating Data of Technical and Scientific, Medical and Trade Book Publishers, 1982	54

Table 4.1:	Sci-Tech and Medical Magazines and Journals, by Subscription and Advertising Revenue, 1982	73
Table 4.2:	Total Estimated Revenue from Advertising and Subscriptions of 25 Leading Technical, Scientific and Medical Magazines and Journals, 1982	74
Table 4.3:	Estimated Revenue of 15 Leading Publishers of Technical, Scientific and Medical Magazines and Journals, 1980	75
Table 4.4:	Cost-Per-Thousand of Selected Medical Magazines	79
Table 4.5:	Wholesale Price Index of Paper, 1973-1983	81
Table 4.6:	Revenue and Expense Model for Controlled-Circulation Medical Magazines Compared With Consumer Magazines	82
Table 4.7:	Revenue and Expense Model for a Commercially Published Journal in the Basic Sciences	96
Table 5.1	Number of U.S. Technical, Scientific and Medical Newsletters Listed in *The Newsletter Yearbook Directory*, by Subject Category, 1983	110
Table 5.2:	Leading TSM Newsletter Publishers, 1980	112
Table 5.3:	Revenue and Expenses for a Weekly Newsletter Priced at $175 Annually, by Circulation and Renewal Rates	122
Table 6.1:	Number of Unique Items Covered by Members of National Federation of Abstracting and Information Services, Selected Years, 1957-1983	134
Table 6.2:	Revenue of Selected Database Publishers in TSM Field, 1980	135
Table 6.3:	Online Databases Offered by DIALOG Information Services, Inc. and Their Online Connect Time Rates, July 1983	138
Table 6.4:	Factors Influencing Future Growth of Databases	165
Table 7.1:	Estimated Revenues and Pretax Profit Margin of 10 Leading TSM Information Companies, 1980	168
Table 7.2:	Estimated and Projected Revenue of the Technical, Scientific and Medical Information Market, by Segment, 1982 and 1988	171

1

Introduction

Because of the explosion of technical, scientific and medical (TSM) information that has taken place during the last decade or two, many fields of knowledge exist today that simply did not exist 20 years ago; other fields have grown tremendously in importance during this period. As a result of this explosion and because professionals must keep abreast of new developments in their fields, a strong demand has been created for TSM information in a variety of forms.

The TSM information market could be broadly defined to include many types of information products and services (including newspapers and catalogs) on technical, scientific or medical subjects, whether aimed at professionals or lay people. However, this study will employ a much narrower definition and will be concerned only with books, newsletters, loose-leaf services, magazines and journals, and database publishing on TSM subjects directed to professionals engaged in TSM fields.

This definition includes those publications that contain the most specialized information for users in TSM fields; these publications are perhaps the most important to the majority of these users. Although this book briefly touches on books and magazines on TSM subjects intended for laymen, this is done in order to point out trends within an industry and does not represent an effort to provide thorough coverage of those aspects of publishing.

In addition, this volume will not discuss publications that are primarily intended for marketing and management personnel employed in TSM fields, since such materials should be considered to fall within the categories of business or trade books and periodicals. Finally, this study will not differentiate between technical and scientific information but, in keeping with general practice within the industry, will consider these two areas as a unit.

The TSM information market, as defined in this book, is estimated to have totaled over $2.3 billion in 1982. (See Table 2.1, for a breakdown by segments. The figure $2307 million given there has been used to calculate percentages detailed below.) The largest sector of the market is magazine and journal publishing, which totaled $893 million in 1982, or 39% of the total TSM information market. Although the size of a given segment of the magazine industry is usually measured in terms of advertising revenue only, many journals, especially those in the scientific-technical (sci-tech) category and in small medical specialties, have little or no advertising revenue. Therefore, this book includes both advertising and subscription revenues in its estimates of the size of the market for TSM magazines and journals. Many medical magazines have controlled circulation, i.e., they are distributed at no charge to their recipients; moreover, many journals sponsored by not-for-profit TSM societies are sent to their members automatically as part of their membership privileges.

The second major segment of the TSM information industry is book publishing, which accounted for $700 million, or 3.3% of the market in 1982. TSM books are defined in this volume as professional books on technical, scientific or medical subjects intended for adult professionals involved in some aspect of these fields. Thus, they are not textbooks, although in the medical field it is difficult, or impossible, for many publishers to distinguish between their textbooks and their books for professionals. Since 1972, TSM books have accounted for only 6% to 8% of total book industry sales, thus constituting a small sector of the book publishing industry as a whole.

The third important part of the TSM information field, database publishing in both hard-copy (print) and online versions, accounted for $660 million or 28.6% of the market in 1982. Although revenues from online services represent less than 20% of the total at this point, they are growing rapidly and, in time, are likely to assume major importance.

Newsletters and loose-leaf services make up the smallest segment of the TSM information market. Together they totaled $54 million in 1982, or 2.4% of the market, with newsletters accounting for $48 million and loose-leaf services for the remainder. The number of newsletters directed to professionals in the TSM industry is relatively small; however, opportunities for growth exist as the volume of knowledge in these fields continues to expand. Similarly, only a handful of loose-leaf services currently serve the TSM field, although it would appear that there is a market for additional services in this area, especially in the sci-tech sector.

THE VOLUME AT HAND

This book examines the present state of the TSM information industry as it is defined above and looks ahead to the next five years and beyond.

Although material has appeared in the trade press regarding various sectors of the TSM information industry and the operations of specific companies, little, if any, literature exists on the business of providing information for professionals in technical, scientific and medical occupations. Yet the amount of available information and the demand for it is steadily increasing. New types of services are being marketed, and computerization has led to the development of new methods of information delivery.

There are problems, too. Some of these, such as rising costs, are common to the entire industry; others, such as increasing postage charges and unauthorized photocopying, affect some sectors more than others.

The various segments of this rapidly changing industry must take the time to consider both their current status and their prospects for the future. This book examines each sector of the industry, describes its economics, discusses new developments and analyzes its opportunities for growth.

Finally, this volume attempts, from an outsider's point of view, to draw some conclusions about the direction in which the industry as a whole appears to be heading, and the challenges it faces in the coming years. Some comparisons are made to earlier analyses, made when this similar data was obtained in 1980 for publication of an industry-only market study of the TSM industry. Information compiled for this book was obtained in 1983 and early 1984.

QUESTIONS TO BE EXAMINED

This book attempts to answer the following questions:

• What is the present size of the TSM market?

• What is the current status of each sector of the TSM information industry?

• How does federal funding of research affect the TSM information industry?

• What effect do shrinking library budgets have on the market for TSM information?

- Are there any differences between medical publishing and sci-tech publishing?

- Will electronic means of information delivery make print services obsolete?

- What is the outlook for each sector of the TSM information industry during the next five years?

LIMITATIONS OF THIS VOLUME

The major limitation of this book stems from the lack of statistical information available on the various segments of the TSM information industry. With the exception of the book segment, no area has compiled detailed statistics about itself. Figures on the advertising revenue of medical magazines and journals are available to subscribers to certain services, and the Information Industry Association has issued reports on the information business as a whole, from which some information on TSM database publishing can be extrapolated. However, in most sectors, executives of major companies had little or no idea of the total sales in their field or, for that matter, of the number of competitors (and this lack of information did not appear to concern them).

Specific difficulties exist with the data in the medical book publishing area. As noted above, many publishers in this sector find it difficult, or impossible, to distinguish between their textbooks and their books for professionals. Although the Association of American Publishers (AAP) has established certain criteria for medical book publishers to follow, it cannot force them to do so. In addition, many publishers point out that a fuzzy line separates scientific books on biological science or physiology, for example, from books on medicine. In the same manner, a book on medical technology may be classified in either the medical or engineering categories. The publishers themselves are often undecided as to how to classify a specific title. Finally, because many of the AAP figures are based on small samples of cooperating publishers, they are not necessarily indicative of the TSM book field as a whole.

With the exception of some available statistics on advertising revenue in medical magazines and journals, little information exists on the size of the TSM magazine and journal sector in terms of the number of publications or in terms of circulation and/or advertising revenue. Although many journal publishers are members of the Professional and Scholarly Division of the AAP, apparently little or no effort has been made to compile statistics similar to those issued annually for the book publishing industry.

Because many TSM information publishers are privately owned or because TSM publishing represents a relatively small part of the operations of a large corporation, it is often difficult to obtain revenue figures by individual publishers. Although some companies in some sectors of the industry were more than willing to share their information and experience with the rest of the industry, many other companies would reveal only the most innocuous data about themselves.

Finally, this volume assumes that most changes in the TSM information industry will be brought about by its members themselves. Its purpose is not to lay down directives for growth but to attempt to put various aspects of the industry into perspective and thus provide a framework within which the industry itself can determine the directions in which to move.

2

Size and Structure of the TSM Information Market

The market for technical, scientific and medical (TSM) information as defined in this book is estimated to have totaled over $2.3 billion in 1982, a 139% increase over the $964 million generated in 1975. About 39% of this figure, or $893 million, was accounted for by advertising and subscription revenue from magazines and journals; TSM books and database publishing accounted for 30% and 29% of the total, respectively; and newsletters and loose-leaf services contributed the smallest portion of revenue, 2.4% or $54 million. Table 2.1 indicates the size of each segment of the market in 1975 and 1982. The following section discusses trends in technical, scientific and medical employment and research, after which each segment of the market will be briefly described.

NUMBER OF PERSONS IN TECHNICAL, SCIENTIFIC AND MEDICAL FIELDS

Ultimately, the size of the TSM information market is determined by the number of persons engaged in each of these fields or preparing to enter them. It appears that not only are these areas already sizable, but that the number of persons involved in them is increasing.

Scientists and Engineers

In 1980, there were 1.50 million engineers and 1.62 million scientists in

Table 2.1 Estimated Size of the Market for Technical, Scientific and Medical Books Information, 1975 and 1982

Segment	1975 Revenue (in millions)	1975 Segment as % of Total	1982 Revenue (in millions)	1982 Segment as % of Total	Percent Increase 1975-1982
Magazines and journals (advertising and subscription revenue)	$459	47.6%	$893	38.7%	94.6%
Technical, scientific and medical books	259	26.9	700	30.3	170.3
Database publishing (hard copy and online)	214	22.2	660	28.6	208.4
Newsletters	30	3.1	48	2.1	60.0
Loose-leaf services	2	0.2	6	0.3	200.0
Total	$964	100.0%	$2307	100.0%	139.3

Note: Discrepancies in totals are due to rounding.
Sources: Books: Association of American Publishers; all other estimates: Knowledge Industry Publications, Inc.

the United States. The number of scientists has grown faster than the number of engineers; during the period, 1976-1980, the number of scientists rose 28.4%, compared to a 24.0% increase in engineers. Atmospheric scientists, computer specialists and biologists enjoyed the fastest growth during this period, while medical scientists and social scientists decreased in number, and oceanographers remained the same. (See Table 2.2.)

Table 2.2 Scientists by Field of Specialization, and Engineers, 1976 and 1980

Field of Specialization	1976	1980	Percent Change 1976-1980
	(in thousands)		
Physical scientists	224	262	+17.0
Chemists	149	171	+14.8
Physicists/astronomers	61	68	+11.5
Other	13	23	+77.0
Computer specialists	210	355	+69.0
Environmental scientists	71	103	+45.1
Earth scientists	59	80	+35.6
Oceanographers	3	3	—
Atmospheric scientists	9	19	+111.0
Life scientists	298	405	+35.9
Biological scientists	141	206	+46.1
Agricultural scientists	108	154	+42.6
Medical scientists	49	45	− 8.2
Psychologists	118	133	+12.7
Mathematical scientists	96	127	+32.3
Social scientists	241	230	−4.6
Total Engineers	1207	1497	+24.0
Total Scientists	1258	1615	+28.4
Total	2465	3111	+26.2

Note: Discrepancies in totals are due to rounding.
Source: U.S. National Science Foundation.

College Enrollment

The number of scientists and engineers entering the marketplace, as well as the number of these professionals with advanced training, is also increasing, a factor which, in turn, will lead to an increased demand for information.

From 1972 to 1980 college enrollment in the major fields of biological sciences, engineering and the physical sciences increased 8.9%, 73.7% and 11.5%, respectively, to reach a total enrollment of nearly 1.1 million students in these fields. (See Table 2.3.)

Table 2.3 College Enrollment in Science and Engineering Curricula, 1972, 1974, 1978 and 1980 (in thousands)

Field of Study	1972	1974	1978	1980	Percent Increase 1972-1980
Biological sciences	257	327	303	280	8.9%
Engineering	357	410	565	620	73.7
Physical sciences	157	134	193	175	11.5
Total	771	871	1,061	1,075	39.4%

Source: 1972-1978: U.S. Dept. of Commerce, Bureau of the Census; 1980: U.S. Dept. of Education, National Center for Education Statistics.

Table 2.4 indicates the number of earned degrees conferred in the sciences in 1979-1980 compared with 1972. With the exception of zoology, physics and psychology, in which fewer bachelor's degrees were awarded, all categories showed increases; geology and biology had increases of 76.0% and 20.5%, respectively. In 1979-1980, some 87,600 engineering degrees were conferred, of which 68,900 were bachelor's degrees.

Physicians and Other Health Professionals

The number of physicians, dentists and nurses has been increasing steadily over the past three decades.

Physicians

In 1980, there were 487,000 physicians in the United States, compared to only 233,000 in 1950, a 109.0% increase. The number of medical schools also increased during this period, as did the number of medical students

Table 2.4 Earned Degrees Conferred in the Sciences, 1972 and 1979-1980

Subject	Bachelor's 1972 (in thousands)	Bachelor's 1979-1980 (in thousands)	Percent Change 1972-1979-1980	Master's 1979-1980	PhD. 1979-1980
Biological sciences[1]	37.6	46.4	+23.4%	6510	3636
Biology	27.8	33.5	+20.5	2911	718
Zoology	5.2	3.7	−28.8	431	245
Engineering	51.5	68.9	+33.8	16,243	2507
Physical sciences[1]	20.9	23.4	+12.0	5219	3089
Chemistry	10.7	11.2	+4.7	1615	1413
Physics	4.6	3.3	−28.3	1177	818
Geology	2.5	4.4	+76.0	1192	260
Psychology	43.4	42.0	−3.2	7806	2768

[1]Total includes subject categories not individually listed.
Source: U.S. Dept. of Education, National Center for Education Statistics.

and annual medical school graduates. In 1980, there were 140 medical and osteopathic schools in the United States, having 68,300 students and graduating 16,200 students; these figures stand in comparison to the 85 schools existent in 1950, having 26,900 students and 5900 graduates. (See Table 2.5.)

The number of physicians in both medical specialties and general practice increased from 1970 to 1980. (See Table 2.6.) The fastest growth occurred in the fields of internal medicine, anesthesiology and pediatrics. The number of internists rose 70.6%, from 41,900 in 1970 to 71,500 in 1980; the number of anesthesiologists rose 58.4%, from 10,100 in 1970 to 16,000 in 1980; and the number of pediatricians increased 58.1% from 17,900 in 1970 to 28,300 in 1980.

According to the American Medical Association, of the 376,500 physicians involved in patient care in 1980, 272,000 were office-based, 42,500 were hospital-based full time, and 62,000 were interns and residents. Another 38,400 doctors were involved in teaching, administration, research and other professional pursuits.

The U.S. Department of Health, Education and Welfare stated that in 1980, California had the greatest number of doctors, 54,082 or 13.1% of all U.S. doctors, followed by New York, with 46,808; Pennsylvania, with 22,098; Texas, with 21,531; and Illinois, with 20,885 physicians (see Table 2.7).

Table 2.5 Number of Physicians, Dentists and Nurses in the U.S. and Schools for Same, Selected Years, 1950 to 1980

Health Professionals and Schools	1950	1955	1960	1965	1970	1975	1977	1980	Percent Increase 1950-1980
Physicians (in thousands)	233	255	275	305	348	409	438	487	109.0%
Doctors of medicine (in thousands)	220	242	260	292	334	394	421	468	112.7
Doctors of osteopathy	13	14	14	13	14	15	17	19	46.2
Medical and osteopathic schools	85	87	91	93	107	123	126	140	64.7
Students (in thousands)	27	30	32	34	40	57	62	68	151.9
Graduates	6	7	8	8	9	13	14	16	166.7
Newly licensed physicians	NA	NA	8,030	9,147	11,032	16,859	18,175	18,200	141.5[1]
Dentists (in thousands)	87	95	103	109	116	NA	133	141	62.1
Dental schools	41	43	47	49	53	59	59	60	46.3
Students (in thousands)	12	13	14	14	16	20	21	22	83.3
Graduates	3	3	3	3	4	5	5	5	66.7
Nurses (active-registered) (in thousands)	375	430	540	613	700	906	1,011	1,119	198.4
Nursing schools	1,203	1,139	1,119	1,153	1,328	1,360	1,337	1,360	13.1
Students (in thousands)	99	108	115	130	151	244	247	235	137.4
Graduates	26	29	30	35	44	75	78	76	192.3

[1]Percentage given is for 1960 to 1980.
Note: Discrepancies in totals for physicians category are due to rounding.
Sources: 1950 to 1975: U.S. Dept. of Commerce; 1977 to 1980: U.S. Dept. of Education, National Center for Health Statistics.

Table 2.6 Physicians by Specialty, 1970, 1975 and 1980.

Specialty	1970	1975	1980	Percent Change 1970-1980
Total[1]	334,000	393,700	467,700	+40.0
General practice	57,900	54,600	60,000	+3.6
Medical[2]	77,200	95,100	125,800	+63.0
Internal medicine	41,900	54,300	71,500	+70.6
Pediatrics	17,900	21,700	28,300	+58.1
Surgical[2]	86,000	96,000	110,800	+28.8
General surgery	29,800	31,600	34,000	+14.1
Obstetrics/gynecology	18,900	21,700	26,300	+39.2
Ophthalmology	9,900	11,100	13,000	+31.3
Orthopedic	9,600	11,400	14,000	+45.8
Other[2]	89,600	94,600	118,300	+32.0
Anesthesiology	10,100	12,900	16,000	+58.4
Psychiatry	21,100	23,900	27,500	+30.3
Pathology	10,300	11,700	13,400	+30.1
Radiology	10,500	11,500	11,700	+11.4

[1]Includes physicians who are inactive, not classified or with address unknown.
[2]Includes specialists not shown separately.
Source: American Medical Association.

Nurses

The nursing profession has shown the fastest growth of the three major health professions. The number of active registered nurses in the United States rose 198.4% during the 1950-1980 period, climbing from 375,000 in 1950 to over 1.1 million in 1980. In 1980 there were 1360 nursing schools with 235,000 students and 76,000 graduates, compared to the 1950 figures of 1203 schools having 99,000 students and 26,000 graduates. (See Table 2.5.)

Other Health Professions

The number of persons employed in other health professions has also increased. Among those occupations showing large increases from 1975 to 1981 were therapists and dietitians, health aides and trainees and clinical laboratory technicians. In 1981 there were 314,000 physical/speech therapists and dietitians, 317,000 health aides and trainees and 276,000 clinical laboratory technicians. (See Table 2.8.)

Table 2.7 U.S. Physicians and Dentists,[1] by State, 1980

State	Active Physicians Number	Percent of Total	Active Dentists Number	Percent of Total
Total	413,692	100.0%	121,240	100.0%
Alabama	4856	1.2	1380	1.1
Alaska	491	0.1	214	0.2
Arizona	4814	1.2	1212	1.0
Arkansas	2772	0.7	793	0.7
California	54,082	13.1	14,346	11.8
Colorado	5664	1.4	1743	1.4
Connecticut	7730	1.9	2290	1.9
Delaware	949	0.2	261	0.2
District of Columbia	3474	0.8	562	0.5
Florida	17,479	4.2	4578	3.8
Georgia	7728	1.9	2142	1.8
Hawaii	1885	0.5	599	0.5
Idaho	1007	0.2	476	0.4
Illinois	20,885	5.0	6214	5.1
Indiana	7022	1.7	2370	2.0
Iowa	3657	0.9	1497	1.2
Kansas	3668	0.9	1095	0.9
Kentucky	4820	1.2	1584	1.3
Louisiana	6501	1.6	1669	1.4
Maine	1680	0.4	505	0.4
Maryland	11,210	2.7	2500	2.1
Massachusetts	15,564	3.8	4079	3.4
Michigan	14,626	3.5	5085	4.2
Minnesota	7718	1.9	2588	2.1
Mississippi	2664	0.6	786	0.6
Missouri	7979	1.9	2404	2.0
Montana	1040	0.3	467	0.4
Nebraska	2319	0.6	985	0.8
Nevada	1097	0.3	353	0.3
New Hampshire	1490	0.4	482	0.4
New Jersey	13,937	3.4	4860	4.0
New Mexico	1972	0.5	558	0.5
New York	46,808	11.3	12,841	10.6
North Carolina	8874	2.1	2203	1.8

Table 2.7 U.S. Physicians and Dentists,[1] by State, 1980 (continued)

State	Active Physicians Number	Percent of Total	Active Dentists Number	Percent of Total
North Dakota	884	0.2	302	0.2
Ohio	17,458	4.2	5337	4.4
Oklahoma	3850	0.9	1237	1.0
Oregon	4760	1.2	1779	1.5
Pennsylvania	22,098	5.3	6664	5.5
Rhode Island	1988	0.5	522	0.4
South Carolina	4129	1.0	1086	0.9
South Dakota	766	0.2	309	0.3
Tennessee	7169	1.7	2164	1.8
Texas	21,531	5.2	5848	4.8
Utah	2373	0.6	917	0.8
Vermont	1087	0.3	293	0.2
Virginia	9154	2.2	2549	2.1
Washington	7381	1.8	2683	2.2
West Virginia	2610	0.6	753	0.6
Wisconsin	7462	1.8	2850	2.4
Wyoming	530	0.1	226	0.2

[1]Excludes doctors of osteopathy, federal physicians and dentists and physicians with addresses unknown.
Note: Discrepancies in totals are due to rounding.
Source: U.S. Dept. of Health, Education and Welfare, National Center for Health Statistics.

RESEARCH AND HEALTH EXPENDITURES

Other factors that affect the market for TSM information include the size of the outlays for scientific research and the volume of health-related expenditures. The size of outlays for research, of course, has a direct relationship to the volume of research results available for publication. Research grants often also include funds to pay for publishing results.

From 1972 to 1982, outlays for scientific research and development more than doubled, rising from $28.5 billion in 1972 to an estimated $77.3 billion in 1982. The proportion of federally funded expenditures declined steadily during this period, from 56% of the total in 1972 to 47% in 1981 and 1982. Table 2.9 indicates the size of outlays on basic research, applied research and development from 1972 through 1982 and the percentage of these funds federally contributed.

Table 2.8 Persons Employed in Selected Health Occupations, 1975 and 1981[1] (in thousands)

Occupation	1975	1981	Percent Increase 1975-1981
Pharmacists	122	152	24.6%
Physical/speech therapists and dietitians	197	314	59.4
Health administrators	154	219	42.2
Health technologists and technicians	406	643	58.4
Clinical laboratory	181	276	52.5
Radiology	80	104	30.0
Other	145	263	81.4
Health service[2]	1734	1995	15.1
Health aides and trainees[3]	222	317	42.8
Nursing aides[4]	1009	1131	12.1
Practical nurses	374	403	7.8

[1]Includes people 16 years old and over.
[2]Includes other occupations not shown separately.
[3]Excludes nursing.
[4]Includes orderlies and attendants.
Note: Discrepancies in totals are due to rounding.
Source: U.S. Dept. of Labor, Bureau of Labor Statistics.

Table 2.9 Outlays for Scientific Research and Development, 1972-1982

Year	Total Expenditures (in billions)	Percent of Expenditures Federally Funded
1972	$28.5	56%
1973	30.7	53
1974	32.9	51
1975	35.2	51
1976	39.0	51
1977	43.0	51
1978	48.3	50
1979	55.0	49
1980	62.2	48
1981	69.8	47
1982[1]	77.3	47

Percent Increase in Total Expenditures, 1972-1982: 171.2%

[1]Estimate.
Source: U.S. National Science Foundation.

Total expenditures on health increased 331.8% from 1970 through 1982 from $74.7 billion in 1970 to $322.4 billion in 1982. Expenditures on medical research increased at a slower pace, rising from close to $2.0 billion in 1970 to $5.9 billion in 1982, a 199.0% increase. Contrary to the situation experienced by research as a whole, the proportion of publicly funded expenditures for medical research crept up steadily during this period, from 89% of total national health expenditures in 1970 to 94.3% in 1982. (See Table 2.10.)

Table 2.10 Total National Health Expenditures on Medical Research, 1970 and 1975-1982 (in millions)

Year	Expenditures Total	Medical Research	Publicly Funded Medical Research as Percent of Total Medical Research
1970	$ 74,663	$1,969	89.0%
1975	132,720	3,335	92.1
1976	149,655	3,701	92.8
1977	169,248	3,919	93.0
1978	189,312	4,444	93.7
1979	214,962	4,785	93.7
1980	248,967	5,328	94.0
1981	286,616	5,653	94.0
1982	322,392	5,888	94.3
Percent Increase, 1970-1982:	331.8%	199.0%	

Source: U.S. Dept. of Health and Human Services, Health Care Financing Administration.

Books

TSM book publishing, together with business and other professional book publishing, comprises the professional publishing category as defined by the Association of American Publishers (AAP).

AAP defines professional books as books directed to professional people and specifically related to their work. Within the professional book category, technical and scientific books deal with subjects in the physical, biological, earth and social sciences, as well as technology, engineering and the trades. The audience for these books is composed of practicing and research scientists, engineers, architects, technicians, mechanics and teachers in these and allied fields. Medical books are directed not only to physicians but also to nurses, dentists, hospital administrators, veterinarians, pharmacists and personnel in allied health fields.

For the purposes of this volume a technical, scientific or medical book will be defined as a professional book on a technical, scientific or medical subject intended for adult professionals involved in some aspect of these fields. It is a nonfiction title that imparts new and advanced information, enabling readers to become more proficient in their careers. AAP figures indicate that sales of TSM books totaled $699.9 million in 1982.

Technical and Scientific Books

Annual figures compiled by the AAP indicate that sales of scientific and technical (sci-tech) books totaled $431.4 million and accounted for 5.4% of total book industry sales in 1982. Sales of sci-tech books have grown at a rate much faster than that of the book industry as a whole during the 1970s and early 1980s.

In 1982, 5452 sci-tech titles were published. Since 1970 technical titles have accounted for an increasing share of sci-tech titles, rising from 32.6% of the combined total in 1970 to 42.7% of the total in 1982.

Prices of hardcover sci-tech books are higher on the average than those of the book industry as a whole. In 1982, the average prices of scientific and technical books were $44.44 and $40.65 respectively, compared with an industry-wide average of $30.34. The combined prices of hardcover sci-tech titles increased at a faster pace during the 1970s and early 1980s than the prices of items in the Consumer Price Index.

Six companies—John Wiley & Sons, McGraw-Hill Book Co., Academic Press, Prentice-Hall, Plenum Publishing Corp., and Van Nostrand Reinhold—accounted for nearly one-third of all sci-tech book volume in 1980, with the remainder divided among other sci-tech book publishers, trade publishers, university presses and professional societies. (In 1982 these companies accounted for 32.7% of sci-tech book volume.)

According to AAP figures, the most important customers for books in the sci-tech category in 1982 were retail stores, wholesalers and jobbers, individuals who made their purchases by mail, and libraries and institutions. International markets are a major growth opportunity for sci-tech publishers. In 1982, the dollar value of U.S. exports of technical, scientific and other professional books totaled $118.5 million.

Medical Books

Until a few years ago, there were only 15 medical book publishers in the United States. Currently, however, according to the American Medical Publishers Association, there are about 35 to 40 major U.S. medical publishers, plus more than 100 publishers who produce one to three books a year that cross over into medicine. There are also many foreign publishers that market medical titles in the United States, some of which are published here.

AAP figures indicate that sales of medical books totaled $268.5 million and accounted for 3.4% of total book industry sales in 1982. During the 1970s, sales of medical books more than tripled and led all sectors of professional book publishing in their rate of growth.

In 1982, 3229 medical titles were published. The number of medical titles published annually has more than doubled during the 1970s, with over half of the increase taking place since 1975. The number of medical titles published in 1982 accounted for 6.9% of all book titles published in that year.

In 1982, the average price of a hardcover medical book was $38.88, compared to an industry-wide average of $30.34. Prices of hardcover medical books increased at a slower pace during the 1970s and early 1980s than prices of items in the Consumer Price Index.

Eight companies—W.B. Saunders & Co., The C.V. Mosby Co., Harper & Row, Publishers, Inc., Year Book Medical Publishers, Springhouse Corp., McGraw-Hill Book Co., The Williams & Wilkins Co., and Little, Brown & Co.—accounted for more than 60% of all medical book revenue in 1980 with the remainder primarily divided between university presses and other medical book publishers.

According to AAP figures, the most important customers for medical titles in 1982 were retail stores, individuals who purchased their books by mail or through salesmen and wholesalers and jobbers. Nearly one-third of the sales of these books were direct from the publisher to the final consumer by mail or through a salesman.

International markets are an important source of sales to the medical publisher. According to the AAP, 11.4% of medical book sales in 1982 were to areas outside the United States and Canada. Industry experts feel this figure is too low, however, and claim that about 25% to 33% of the sales of most American medical publishers are to overseas customers, with the English-speaking countries and Japan said to be the most important.

Magazines and Journals

Revenues from magazine and journal publishing in the TSM field totaled an estimated $893 million in 1982. There are several distinct differences between magazines and journals. A journal is usually a scholarly publication devoted to the first announcement of research or to original works written by the persons who conducted the research.

Magazines, on the other hand, provide an overview of a subject and contain news and applications of research.

The basic difference between magazines and journals, however, is that of peer review, whereby a submitted article is reviewed by one or more individuals in the field to decide if it is suitable for publication in a specific journal. In the medical publishing field, the terms "magazine" and "journal" are often used interchangeably, but true journals involve peer review and subscription charge to the readers.

There are relatively few magazines devoted to professionals in the sci-tech field. The actual number, in fact, is probably less than 100. The important magazines in this sector are those published by three professional nonprofit associations—The Institute of Electrical and Electronic Engineers (IEEE), the American Chemical Society and the American Institute of Physics (AIP)—and include *IEEE Spectrum, Chemical & Engineering News* and *Physics Today.*

Estimates of the number of sci-tech journals published in the United States range as high as 18,000 to 20,000. It is more likely, however, that in 1982 there were between 4000 and 5000 sci-tech journals published in the United States. It is extremely difficult, if not impossible, to obtain reliable separate estimates of the number of U.S.-published medical magazines and journals, but it is probable that the number of such periodicals— excluding local, county and state publications—is between 1200 and 3000.

Revenue from subscriptions to TSM journals is estimated to have totaled about $600 million in 1982, with medical journals accounting for about $200 million and sci-tech publications for the remaining $400 million. Since the majority of medical magazines have controlled circulation, their subscription revenue is practically nil. Subscription revenue from the less than 100 sci-tech magazines is estimated at $12 to $18 million. Thus, total subscription revenue from TSM magazines and journals probably reached about $618 million in 1982.

Advertising revenue of sci-tech journals and magazines is small, probably amounting to about $25 million. Advertising revenue of medical magazines and journals, on the other hand, is 10 times that amount, totaling about $250 million.

The five leading U.S. publishers of TSM magazines and journals in terms of 1980 revenue were the Medical Economics Co., Academic Press, the American Medical Association, the American Institute of Physics and McGraw-Hill Publications Co. The 15 leading U.S. publishers of TSM magazines and journals in 1980 accounted for 26.9% of total estimated revenue from TSM journals and magazines.

The top five TSM magazines in terms of total 1982 revenues were *New England Journal of Medicine, Medical Economics, Machine Design,*

Science and *Nursing '82*. The 25 leading TSM magazines and journals accounted for 26.2% of estimated total industry revenue in 1982. About 82% of their revenue was derived from advertising, while subscription revenue accounted for the remaining 18%. Most medical magazines have little or no international circulation. Foreign subscriptions to TSM journals, however, generally account for 30% to 50% of the total.

Newsletters

A newsletter is a concise periodical directed to a special-interest group; it is sold by subscription only and ordinarily contains no advertising. Newsletters thus charge readers the entire cost of publication, unlike magazines which are able to charge their readers only a fraction of their publishing costs.

A newsletter usually carries up-to-the-minute concise information on current developments in a field. This is in contrast to a journal which contains in-depth scholarly papers on research findings in a specific area, which have been reviewed before publication by a panel of experts in the field.

The fourth edition of *The Newsletter Yearbook Directory* lists 420 newsletters that can be classified as TSM letters, a small portion of the 5000 newsletters K.I.P.I. estimated were in existence in 1981. TSM newsletters had estimated revenues of $48 million in 1982.

Newsletters in the TSM category have circulations ranging from several hundred copies to a high of 135,000 copies for *The Medical Letter*; the majority, however, have circulations of less than 5000 copies. A conservative estimate of the 1983 circulation of all TSM letters would be about 600,000 copies. The Medical Letter, McGraw-Hill Publications Co. and M.J. Powers & Co. are among the largest publishers of TSM newsletters in terms of revenue.

Loose-Leaf Services

A loose-leaf reference service is simply a reference volume or volumes on a specific topic presented in a binder so that it may be updated on a regular basis. The services are meant to be comprehensive reference sources but differ from textbooks in that their information is always current.

Few such services exist in the scientific and technical area. Only three major companies are publishing in the medical sector, while several services, such as those published by Aspen Systems Corp., exist in the health-law field. The loose-leaf service area is the smallest sector of the

TSM information service market, accounting for an estimated $6 million of revenue.

Harper & Row, with 10 medical services is by far the major company in the TSM loose-leaf service field. Other major publishers in the field include Scientific American, which publishes *Scientific American Medicine*, a two-volume service, and Futura Publishing Co., Inc., which has published six volumes of *Modern Technics in Surgery*, a projected 10-volume service.

Database Publishing: Print and Online

A database is an organized collection of data, usually in machine-readable form. In order to be considered a database, however, a product must have several key characteristics, among them comprehensiveness, in-depth indexing and ease of retrieval of specific items. In addition, a database product is intended for reference use rather than for casual reading.

A database may be in printed form (hard copy), computerized (online), or both. If the customer has direct access to the computerized database through a terminal, the database is termed "online"; the majority of such databases are derived from printed services. The online database business originated with scientific and technical files, each of which generally covers a particular branch of science or technology and consists of bibliographic citations and abstracts of scientific journal articles, research reports, conference proceedings, monographs, and so on.

In 1982 the market for hard-copy and online TSM database publishing was estimated at $660 million, of which $125 million was online and $535 million was print. (These figures include databases published by not-for-profit organizations and government agencies and also include revenues of database vendors.) It is likely that about 400 organizations (including commercial and not-for-profit organizations) are engaged in TSM database publishing. In early 1984 there were an estimated 175 bibliographic, textual or full-text databases in the TSM area produced in the United States.

Among the leaders in their respective sectors of the TSM field are Chemical Abstracts Service, a division of the American Chemical Society; the National Library of Medicine; Engineering Information Inc.; and the Institute for Scientific Information. Revenues of these organizations ranged from $3 million to $36 million in 1980, yet each is a leader in its particular segment of the TSM database spectrum.

Online databases are made available to users through information vendors that publicly sell their own or other producers' databases on time-sharing computer systems. The largest vendor, with over 180 databases, is DIALOG Information Services, Inc., a subsidiary of Lockheed Corporation. Other leading U.S. database vendors include Bibliographic Retrieval Services (BRS), the National Library of Medicine (NLM) and System Development Corporation (SDC).

International sales are important in both the print and online sectors of the TSM database market. Many of the major producers of print databases find that a large part of their sales are to foreign customers, and online databases are also marketed abroad by database vendors.

3

Books

Technical, scientific and medical (TSM) book publishing is one of the principal categories of professional book publishing, as defined by the Association of American Publishers (AAP).

DEFINITION AND SCOPE OF TSM BOOKS

The AAP defines professional books as books directed to professional people and specifically related to their work. Another useful definition is that provided by Harry R. Most in a 1977 article in *Publishers Weekly*.[1] Most defined professional publishing as "the creation of books to satisfy the continuing educational needs of the practicing professional after he or she has finished using textbooks...."

Within the professional book category, the AAP states that technical and scientific books deal with subjects in the physical, biological, earth and social sciences, as well as technology, engineering and the trades. Their audience is composed of practicing and research scientists, engineers, architects, technicians, mechanics and teachers in these and allied fields. Medical books are directed not only to physicians but also to nurses, dentists, hospital administrators, veterinarians, pharmacists and personnel in allied health fields.

In this book, a technical, scientific or medical book is defined as a book on a technical, scientific or medical subject intended for adult professionals involved in some aspect of these fields. Such a book does not aim to impart information on these subjects to the general public, although in rare cases a

---

[1] "Today's Best Book Profits Are In Professional Publishing," March 21, 1977, p. 39.

technical book becomes a bestseller; e.g., Masters' and Johnson's *Human Sexual Response* was published by the medical division of Little, Brown at a short discount. Few publishers in the scientific-technical (sci-tech) field draw a sharp distinction between their scientific and technical titles, and the AAP has no hard and fast definitions for these categories. This chapter will follow book industry practice and consider scientific and technical publishing as a unit.

Distribution Problems

In considering sales figures for books in the TSM field, it should be noted that many publishers in the medical area find it difficult, or impossible, to distinguish between their textbooks and their books for professionals. In addition, industry spokesmen point out that a fuzzy line separates books on biological science or physiology from books on medicine; in the same way, a book on medical technology may be classified in either the medical or engineering categories. Thus, publishers themselves are often undecided as to how to categorize a specific title.

A title in the medical field may also have a textual or a clinical orientation. A title with a textual orientation could be used as a text by residents and at the same time be read by practitioners to increase their knowledge. Thus, in some instances, this book could be considered a textbook. A title with a clinical orientation contains more advanced information and is intended for the practicing professional.

Many industry spokesmen say there is no way to exclude textbooks from medical book figures. Moreover, nursing titles, which are mostly textbooks, are generally included in medical book sales. Although the AAP has established certain criteria, it cannot force publishers to follow them. Clearly, some books are used both as texts and as books for practitioners. Doctors living near university medical bookstores purchase titles they desire from this source. For example, McGraw-Hill is thought to sell 62,000 to 65,000 copies of *Harrisons' Principles of Internal Medicine* every four years, but one-half to two-thirds of its sales are said to be to practitioners. This type of sales pattern, incidentally, reduces the risk of textbook publishing because the professional market can always be counted on for extra sales.

SIZE OF THE TSM BOOK MARKET

Sales

Annual figures compiled by the AAP indicate that sales of sci-tech books more than tripled during the last 10 years, rising from $131.8 million in 1972 to $431.4 million in 1982, a 227.3% increase. Sales of medical books more than quadrupled during this period, rising from $57.0 million in 1972 to $268.5 million in 1982, a 371.1% increase. Within the professional book area, medical books led all categories in their rate of growth and accounted for some 2% to 3% of book industry sales during this period. Sci-tech books were second in their rate of growth and accounted for 4% to 5% of total industry sales during this period. Sales of the book industry as a whole increased 164.1% from 1972 to 1982, rising from $3017.8 million in 1972 to $7971.5 million in 1982. (See Table 3.1).

There are several reasons for rapid increases in the sales of sci-tech and medical titles: Neither the medical nor the sci-tech publishing field is greatly affected by economic fluctuations. Purchasers are professionals who must buy these books in order to be well informed and to succeed in their professions. Although prices are relatively high, there is little price resistance because the books are considered necessities and, in the sci-tech field, are often purchased for an individual by his or her employer. To the extent that purchases are made by libraries and academic institutions, however, there has been a distinct slowdown in sales since the late 1970s.

In TSM publishing, as in other areas, the "twigging" phenomenon leads to growth. The term twigging, coined by Curtis Benjamin, former president and chairman of McGraw-Hill, describes the increasingly narrow specialization brought about both by the refinement of research and by the knowledge explosion. As various medical and scientific branches grow more numerous, or "twig," and the twigs, in turn, do twigging of their own, the number of subjects for books grows proportionately. (The other side of the coin, however, is that the audience for an individual book tends to shrink, and some books with extremely narrow appeal can no longer be published profitably.)

Because of the explosion of technical, scientific and medical knowledge, many fields of interest exist today that did not exist 25 years ago, while others have grown in importance. Since professionals must keep abreast of new developments in their fields, a demand for books is created.

In addition, the number of engineers, scientists, and physicians and other health professionals is increasing. From 1974 to 1980, the number of engineers rose by 185,000 or 14%, and the number of scientists by 297,000 or 25%. From 1970 to 1980, the number of physicians rose by 139,000 or 39.9%; the number of dentists by 25,000 or 21.6%; and the number of nurses by 419,000 or 59.9%. Thus, larger numbers of professionals in the

Table 3.1 Sales of Professional Books, Technical and Scientific Books, Medical Books and Total Book Industry Sales, 1972-1982
(in millions)

Year	Professional Books Dollar Sales	Professional Books Annual % Increase	Technical and Scientific Books Dollar Sales	Technical and Scientific Books Annual % Increase	Medical Books Dollar Sales	Medical Books Annual % Increase	Total Industry Dollar Sales	Total Industry Annual % Increase	Sales of TSM Books as % of Industry Sales Technical and Scientific	Sales of TSM Books as % of Industry Sales Medical
1972	$ 381.0	7.9%	$131.8	7.8%	$ 57.0	8.8%	$3017.8	3.4%	4.4%	1.9%
1973	405.4	6.4	138.4	5.0	60.8	6.7	3213.6	6.5	4.3	1.9
1974	466.3	15.0	158.3	14.4	71.7	17.9	3569.9	11.1	4.4	2.0
1975	501.2	7.5	175.5	10.9	83.4	16.3	3850.7	7.9	4.6	2.2
1976	559.0	11.5	195.2	11.2	97.0	16.3	4185.2	8.7	4.7	2.3
1977	698.2	24.9	249.3	27.7	162.6	67.6	5142.2	22.9	4.8	3.2
1978	804.6	15.2	277.5	11.3	193.8	19.2	5792.5	12.6	4.8	3.3
1979	885.1	10.0	301.1	8.5	214.0	10.4	6332.2	9.3	4.8	3.4
1980	999.1	12.9	334.8	11.2	239.9	12.1	7039.4	11.2	4.8	3.4
1981	1140.7	14.2	391.1	16.8	256.9	7.1	7665.1	8.9	4.8	3.4
1982	1230.5	7.9	431.4	10.3	268.5	4.5	7971.5	4.0	4.8	3.4
% Increase	223.0%		227.3%		371.1%		164.1%			

Source: Association of American Publishers.

sci-tech and medical areas create an expanding demand for books in their fields of interest.

To some extent, government and private funding of research also influences sales of medical and sci-tech books. For example, public programs in energy and environmental science have been accelerated recently. Publishers, in turn, are developing new publishing programs to meet the growing demand for information in these fields. In addition, many books are purchased with grant funds or institutional funds, making it easier for publishers to pass along cost increases. Cuts in library, education and research funding all slow the increase in such purchases, however.

Another growth factor is that the world has become the marketplace for high-level sci-tech and medical books. Since the end of World War II, English has been the world's second language and the language of science and medicine. Both medical and sci-tech books have great transportability in their original English and can be translated into many languages. In addition, progress in developing nations has led to a demand for more sci-tech books.

Relationship of the Book Industry to Gross National Product

Sales of sci-tech and medical books, and of the book industry as a whole, have shown a significant relationship to the gross national product (GNP) in the past 10 years. From 1972 through 1974, sales of sci-tech books grew at a slower pace than GNP; from 1975 through 1982 the growth rate of sci-tech book sales exceeded that of the GNP. In 1973, sales of medical books grew at a slower rate than GNP; starting in 1974, however, the growth rate of medical books sales exceeded that of the GNP, and with each succeeding year the gap between the two has widened. Sales of both types of books have also increased at a rate much faster than that of the industry as a whole. (See Table 3.2).

Number of Titles

The number of sci-tech titles published annually since 1970 has ranged from a low of 3499 in 1970 to a peak of 5688 in 1981. In 1982 this number dropped to 5452. Since 1970, technical books have increased their share of titles in the sci-tech category, rising from 32.6% of the combined total in 1970 to 42.7% of the total in 1982. The number of titles in the technical category rose 102.7% from 1970 to 1981, compared to a 43.1% increase in the number of scientific titles during the same period.

The number of medical titles published annually since 1970 has also

Table 3.2 Index of Technical and Scientific Book Sales, Medical Book Sales and Total Industry Sales Compared with Gross National Product, 1972-1982 (in millions). Index (1972 = 100)

Year	Technical and Scientific Books Dollar Sales	Index	Medical Books Dollar Sales	Index	Total Book Industry Dollar Sales	Index	Gross National Product Dollars (in billions)	Index
1972	$131.8	100.0	$ 57.0	100.0	$3017.8	100.0	$1185.9	100.0
1973	138.4	105.0	60.8	106.7	3213.6	106.5	1326.4	111.8
1974	158.3	120.1	71.7	125.8	2569.9	118.3	1434.2	120.9
1975	175.5	133.2	83.4	146.3	3850.7	127.6	1549.2	130.6
1976	195.2	148.1	97.0	170.2	4185.2	138.7	1718.0	144.9
1977	249.3	189.2	162.6	285.3	5142.2	170.4	1918.3	161.8
1978	277.5	210.5	193.8	340.0	5792.5	191.9	2163.9	182.5
1979	301.1	228.5	214.0	375.4	6332.2	209.8	2417.8	203.9
1980	334.8	254.0	239.9	420.9	7039.4	233.3	2631.7	221.9
1981	391.1	296.7	256.9	450.7	7665.1	254.0	2954.1	249.1
1982	431.4	327.3	268.5	471.1	7971.5	264.1	3073.0	259.1

Sources: Book sales: Association of American Publishers; Gross national product: U.S. Dept. of Commerce.

grown, from 1476 titles in 1970 to 3229 titles in 1982, a rise of 118.8%. Since 1970, medical titles have accounted for an increasing proportion of all book titles, rising from 4.1% of the total in 1970 to 6.9% of all titles in 1982. During this period, the total number of book titles published rose 30.1%, from 36,071 in 1970 to 46,935 in 1982 (see Table 3.3 for a summary by five-year periods). It should be kept in mind, however, that although the number of medical titles has increased during the 1970s, with the exception of major books that lack competition, unit sales per title have decreased.

Table 3.3 Trends in Technical, Scientific and Medical Book Titles, 1970-1982

	Average Number of Titles Published Yearly			
	Technical	Scientific	Medical	Total Books
1970-1974	1363	2681	1851	38,525
1975-1979	2023	2968	2749	42,050
1980-1982	2326	3203	3436	46,035
% Increase 1970-1974 to 1980-1982	70.7%	19.5%	85.6%	19.5%

	TSM Books as a Percentage of Total Books		
	Technical and Scientific	Medical	Total TSM
1970	9.7%	4.1%	13.8%
1975	11.8	5.8	17.6
1980	12.9	7.8	20.6
1982	11.6	6.9	18.5

Source: Knowledge Industry Publications, Inc. calculations based on figures from R.R. Bowker.

TYPES OF BOOKS

In addition to ordinary books, TSM publishers—especially those publishing on purely scientific subjects of interest only to researchers—may also produce advances, treatises, series and monographs, all of which are in book form and have the same publishing economies as ordinary TSM books.

Advances

Advances are usually annual publications that cover a broad topic (e.g., energy systems and technology) and contain critical review articles by specialists in the field. These articles cover, criticize and interpret journal articles (not necessarily those of the current year) on a specific topic and deal with developments in the field. For example, Academic Press publishes *Advances in Agronomy* (edited by A.G. Norman) and *Advances in Aquatic Microbiology* (edited by M.R.Droop and H.W. Jannasch). Advances are primarily purchased by libraries but are also bought by individuals.

Treatises

A treatise consists of one or more volumes covering a field, usually a narrow one, in a systematic manner. The volumes are comprehensive and contain in-depth articles on various aspects of the subject, written by the top individuals in the field. Academic Press, for example, publishes *Plant Disease: An Advanced Treatise* (edited by J.G. Horsfall and E.B. Cowling). This publication consists of five volumes: *How Disease Is Managed, How Disease Develops In Populations, How Plants Suffer From Disease, How Pathogens Induce Disease* and *How Plants Defend Themselves*. Ordinarily, a treatise is a library or laboratory item because of its expense; the set referred to above is priced at $229.50.

Series

A series is a group of books on a broad subject in which each individual title deals with a narrow segment. The books are often in textbook form but are written on a higher level for professionals and may be treatises or monographs. One example is the Academic Press Series in Cognition and Perception, edited by Edward C. Carterette and Morton P. Friedman, which currently contains 22 volumes.

Monographs

Monographs, which are especially popular in medical publishing, are highly intensive detailed discussions of very specialized topics. For example, a book might deal with foot surgery, but a monograph would be concerned only with the removal of benign tumors of the big toe. Because of increasing specialization in the medical field, monographs are growing in popularity. Three examples of monographs, all published by Academic

Press, are *Theory of Optimum Aerodynamic Shapes: External Problems in the Aerodynamics of Supersonic, Hypersonic and Free-Molecular Flows* (edited by Angelo Miele), *Stability of Parallel Flow* (by Robert Betchov and William O. Criminale, Jr.) and *Flow Equation for Composite Gases* (by J.M. Burgers).

Leading Publishers of Sci-Tech Books

No exact count is possible of the number of publishers of sci-tech books, but the number is certainly in the hundreds, particularly when associations and professional societies—many of which may issue only a title or two a year—are included. There are 140 companies that are members of AAP's Professional and Scholarly Division and there are 78 members of the Association of University Presses, most of which publish sci-tech books. Many trade publishers, such as Random House, produce an occasional sci-tech title; in addition, a number of European or British companies have American branches that publish sci-tech books in the United States, including Elsevier North-Holland, Springer Verlag New York, Masson, Pergamon Press and Longman.

Top Six Companies

The leading publishers in terms of sci-tech book sales are John Wiley & Sons; McGraw-Hill Book Co.; Academic Press (a subsidiary of Harcourt Brace Jovanovich); Prentice-Hall; Plenum Publishing Corp.; and Van Nostrand Reinhold (a subsidiary of the International Thomson Organisation, Ltd.). In 1980 these six companies accounted for nearly one-third of all sci-tech book volume, with the remainder divided among the sci-tech book publishers, trade publishers, university presses and professional societies. (See Table 4.4.) In 1982 these companies are estimated to have accounted for 32.7% of all sci-tech book volume.

It should be kept in mind that a publisher may not be equally strong in both the scientific and technical areas. McGraw-Hill, for example, is strong in engineering titles, while the strength of Academic Press lies in the pure sciences. A useful classification is that of a professional versus a research publisher. A professional publisher, such as McGraw-Hill, publishes for professional people involved in a specific field. Academic Press and Plenum Press, on the other hand, are primarily research publishers, publishing pure science of interest to scientific researchers. Wiley is both a research and a professional publisher, publishing works intended for both markets. A brief description follows of the activities of each of the six leading publishers in the sci-tech area.

34   TECHNICAL, SCIENTIFIC AND MEDICAL PUBLISHING

Table 3.4 Estimated Revenue of Six Leading Scientific and Technical Book Publishers, 1980

Publisher	Estimated Scientific and Technical Book Revenue (in millions)
John Wiley & Sons	$30[1]
McGraw-Hill Book Co.	26
Academic Press	20
Prentice-Hall	16
Plenum Publishing Corp.	9
Van Nostrand Reinhold	8
Total	$109
Total 1980 sales of scientific and technical books	$334.8
Six leading companies' share of total scientific and technical book revenue	32.6%

[1]Figure given is for fiscal 1980.
Source: Knowledge Industry Publications, Inc.

John Wiley & Sons

Wiley's sales of sci-tech books in fiscal 1980 were estimated at $30 million, or 29% of its net sales of $103 million. In 1982 its sales of sci-tech books were estimated at $38.3 million. The company is predominant in the physics and chemistry markets and is a leader in computer books. It also publishes 29 primary scientific research journals. Wiley also publishes titles in the medical and business fields and is a publisher of undergraduate- and graduate-level college textbooks.

McGraw-Hill

McGraw-Hill Book Co.'s estimated $26 million in sci-tech book sales accounted for about 7% of the company's 1980 sales of $355 million. Its 1982 sales of sci-tech books are estimated at $30.1 million. Although it publishes some pure science titles, most of its books are in the engineering field, and its greatest strength lies in its line of engineering handbooks and in its computer titles. In addition to the approximately 150 sci-tech titles it publishes annually, McGraw-Hill Book Co. publishes medical, law and business books, textbooks, trade books, educational and training materials, and books in other professional areas.

Academic Press

Academic Press, a subsidiary of Harcourt Brace Jovanovich, had estimated 1980 sales of sci-tech books totaling $20 million or 29% of total estimated company sales of $70 million. Academic's 1982 sales of sci-tech books are estimated at $25.0 million. The company publishes advances, treatises, series and monographs in addition to books, textbooks and journals in the fields of science, engineering and other technology, and medicine.

Prentice-Hall

Prentice-Hall's sales of sci-tech titles in 1980 were estimated at $16 million, or 33% of the company's $47.8 million in sales of business and professional books. Titles are geared to professionals in electronics, engineering and computer science. The company also publishes titles in areas such as education, medicine, law and business. In 1982 Prentice Hall's sales of sci-tech books are estimated at $29.3 million.

Plenum Publishing Corp.

Plenum's sales of sci-tech titles were estimated at $9 million in 1980. Its Plenum Press Division publishes scientific, technical and medical titles, including treatises, monographs and other advanced text-reference works, as well as meeting proceedings, works surveying the state of the art in various scientific fields and specialized bibliographies and data compilations. The division also publishes over 60 scientific journals. In 1982 Plenum's sales of sci-tech books remained flat at an estimated $9 million.

Van Nostrand Reinhold

The Professional and Reference Division of Van Nostrand Reinhold (VNR), a subsidiary of the International Thomson Organisation, Ltd. was estimated to have had sales of sci-tech books totaling about $8 million in 1980, 50% of total company sales of $16 million. VNR's 1982 sales of sci-tech books are estimated at $9.4 million. In 1982 VNR established the Scientific and Academic Editions division, which publishes and imports specialized monographs, advanced texts, research and theoretical treatises and symposia in physical, earth, environmental, life and social and behavioral sciences. Together with Wiley and McGraw-Hill, it is one of the three leading publishers of sci-tech encyclopedias.

NUMBER OF MEDICAL PUBLISHERS AND LEADING COMPANIES

Until recent years there were only 15 medical book publishers in the United States. Currently, however, according to the American Medical Publishers Association, there are about 35 to 40 primary, or major, U.S. medical publishers, plus more than 100 publishers who produce one to three books a year that cross over into medicine. (A physics book, for example, may touch on medicine and be marketed to doctors.) There are also many foreign publishers, such as Elsevier North-Holland, that market medical titles in the United States, some of which are published in this country.

The increase in the number of U.S. medical publishers can be attributed to several factors. During the 1970s an information explosion took place in the medical field. The CAT scanner was developed; changes took place in the philosophy of psychiatry; increased information became available on how drugs work, etc. Annual outlays for health care more than tripled. All these trends created publishing opportunities. The medical publishing field also may be a hedge against both recession and inflation. Doctors will buy books in a recession because they regard the information they contain as a necessity. Similarly, because of the physician's need for this material, a publisher can easily pass on cost increases in a period of inflation.

In theory, it is easy to enter the medical publishing field with little investment up front; e.g., by getting the rights to publish symposium proceedings with a limited printing. Small, specialized markets enable the publisher to promote to target audiences at modest cost. But attracting manuscripts from the top authorities in the world means severe competition, and here the tiny undercapitalized publisher is at a disadvantage.

In practice then, medical publishing is highly concentrated; in 1980 the top eight companies (see Table 3.5) accounted for more than 60% of industry revenues. The remainder was divided primarily among university presses and medical book publishers, such as Raven Press and Appleton-Century-Crofts (a subsidiary of Prentice-Hall), and relatively new publishers, such as Futura Press, that choose one or two specialty areas in which to publish clinical monographs marketed to individuals and libraries usually by direct mail.

It should be kept in mind that in this book the term "medical books" also includes nursing, dental, and other titles in the health fields. In addition, because of the difficulty many industry publishers have in differentiating between textbooks and books for clinicians, the totals in Table 3.5 may

Table 3.5 Estimated Revenue of Eight Leading Medical[1]
Book Publishers, 1980

Publisher	Estimated Medical[1] Book Revenue (in millions)
W.B. Saunders & Co.	$ 40
The C.V. Mosby Co.	25
Harper & Row, Publishers, Inc.	20
Year Book Medical Publishers	19
Springhouse Corp.[2]	13
McGraw-Hill Book Co.	12
The William & Wilkins Co.	11
Little, Brown & Co.	9
Total	$149
Total 1980 sales of medical books	$239.9
Eight leading companies' share of total	62.1%

[1]Includes revenue from nursing books and other titles in health fields.
[2]In 1983 Intermed Communications, Inc. changed its name to Springhouse Corp.
Note: Because of the difficulty medical publishers have in differentiating between textbooks and books for practitioners, these figures may include an undetermined amount of textbook revenue.
Source: Knowledge Industry Publications, Inc.

reflect an undetermined amount of textbook sales. A brief description follows of the activities of each of the eight leading publishers in the medical field.

W.B. Saunders Co.

W.B. Saunders Co., a part of the CBS Educational and Professional Publishing Division, claims to be the world's leading health sciences publisher. Its estimated 1980 book sales of $40 million were probably evenly divided between textbooks and books for practitioners. The company publishes medical, nursing, dental, veterinary and allied health titles, including books for medical secretaries; about 20% of its sales are in nursing. Saunders also publishes 24 *Clinics in North America*, a series of hardbound periodicals issued three to six times annually, and one journal, *The American Journal of Otolaryngology*. In spring 1980, it became the first major professional publisher in the United States to enter the trade-publishing field by beginning the publication of health-related titles for the general reader.

The C.V. Mosby Co.

The C.V. Mosby Co., a part of The Times Mirror Co. Professional Publishing Group, claims to be the second largest health sciences publisher in the world and is the leading publisher in the fields of nursing and dentistry. Mosby, which has about 2000 active titles in print and had estimated medical book sales of $25 million in 1980, publishes texts in the medical, nursing, dental and allied health fields in addition to books for practitioners and 19 journals. (A new journal began publication in early 1984.) It also has a small, but growing, operation in college textbooks in the basic sciences, such as biochemistry, and in special education. In 1982 Mosby began publishing books for the general reader on medical topics, and in 1983 it established a software publishing division to develop software products for professionals and students in medicine, nursing, dentistry and allied health.

Harper & Row, Publishers, Inc.

Harper & Row (including its subsidiary, The J.B. Lippincott Co.) publishes medical titles under both the Harper & Row and Lippincott imprints. In addition to its medical book sales, which totaled $20 million in 1980, it publishes 34 journals and several loose-leaf services; about 25% of its titles are in the nursing field.

Year Book Medical Publishers

Year Book, also a part of The Times Mirror Co. Professional Publishing Group, had medical book sales estimated at $19 million in 1980. Year Book publishes 25 yearbooks annually. These books, which constitute one-third of its publishing program and account for 50% to 55% of its sales, are each devoted to a different specialty and are digests of the most significant and relevant literature of the year culled from over 500 journals. The remaining two-thirds of the company's titles are published for clinicians. Year Book publishes only a few textbooks, although it has some titles that are purchased by both students and practitioners. The company also publishes seven periodicals, with each issue devoted exclusively to a single topic of major importance, and two monthly newsletters, *The Year Book of Pediatrics Newsletter* and *The Year Book of Urology Newsletter*.

Springhouse Corp.

Springhouse, formerly Intermed Communications, is the publisher of

Nursing '84, the largest nursing magazine in the United States. The company publishes an annual, *Nurse's Guide to Drugs*, and books on nursing subjects which are marketed as continuity series to *Nursing '84's* 542,000 subscribers; currently Springhouse is marketing three such series. Springhouse's book sales in 1980 were estimated at $13 million. In 1981 its book sales were estimated at $74 million.

McGraw-Hill Book Co.

The Health Professions Division of McGraw-Hill Book Co. publishes 15 to 20 medical books for students and practitioners annually. Most of its books are text-references that can be used in class by students and as references by practitioners. In 1980 its estimated sales were $12 million, of which about $7 million came from books on medical subjects and $5 million from nursing titles. In 1981 nursing books began to be published by the company's college division.

The Williams & Wilkins Co.

The Williams & Wilkins Co., a division of Waverly Press, publishes textbooks and books for practitioners; it claims to be second to Saunders in the medical text market. Its greatest strength is in the field of anatomy. In addition to its books, the company publishes 43 journals. It is the leading commercial publisher of medical society journals and ranks third in terms of the total number of medical journals published. In 1980, its book sales totaled $11 million; in 1982 books accounted for 42% of its publishing revenue, or $12.3 million.

Little, Brown & Co.

Little, Brown, a subsidiary of Time Inc., published 70 titles in the fields of medicine, nursing and allied health in 1983. It is the publisher of Masters' and Johnson's *Human Sexual Response*, one of the few medical titles to hit the best-seller lists. The company, which had estimated medical book sales of $9 million in 1980, also publishes four journals and two hardcover quarterlies.

DISTRIBUTION OF TSM BOOKS

TSM books are sold to retail stores, wholesalers and jobbers, libraries and institutions, and individuals. They are sometimes sold to the college market for textbook use, and they also enjoy sizable international sales.

According to figures compiled by the AAP, in 1982 the most important customers for books in the sci-tech category were retail stores, wholesalers and jobbers, individuals who made their purchases by mail, and libraries and institutions. (See Table 3.6.) The most important customers for medical titles were retail stores, individuals who purchased their books by mail or through salesmen, and wholesalers and jobbers. Nearly one-third of the sales of these books were direct from the publisher to the final consumer by mail or through a salesman.

Retail Store Sales of Scientific and Technical Books

According to the AAP, retail stores accounted for 33.5% of sci-tech book sales in 1982. College bookstores and "other retailers," which includes sci-tech bookstores, accounted for 17.6% of sales, and general bookstores accounted for the remaining 15.7%. (The figure for general bookstores seems high, and may reflect the fact that only 29 professional publishers reported this information to the AAP.) Industry spokesmen say sci-tech bookstores, university and college bookstores and stores that have established a sci-tech section are the most important outlets for sci-tech books.

Of the 19,049 retail book outlets in the United States and regions administered by the U.S. listed in the *American Book Trade Directory—1982*, only 57 are in the science and technology category. An additional 2718 are college stores that may carry some sci-tech titles, depending on the level and extent of their graduate departments.

It is difficult to persuade a general bookstore to carry sci-tech titles for several reasons: the retailer does not understand their contents; the books are more expensive than other titles; they are sold at short discounts; and the retailer may lack sufficient space to store them. Publishers are attempting to encourage general bookstores to carry sci-tech titles by having their salesmen actively promote them when they are calling on a bookstore account. In addition, publishers are encouraging retailers to participate in agency plans and/or cooperative advertising plans, and are providing discounts as described below.

Agency Plans

Under an agency plan a retailer receives a higher discount on a short discount sci-tech title. In return, he usually must agree to the automatic shipment of at least one copy of each new title in a certain number of subject categories. In addition, a minimum initial order and a mininum inventory are normally required.

Table 3.6 Sales of Technical and Scientific Books and Medical Books, by Type of Customer, 1982

Type of Customer	Technical and Scientific	Medical
	(percent of total sales)	
Retail Stores	33.5%	36.7%
General bookstores	15.7	15.0
College bookstores	13.5	21.2
Other retailers	4.1	0.4
Wholesalers and Jobbers	20.5	26.4
Library jobbers	17.7	9.0
All other jobbers	2.8	17.4
Libraries and Institutions	13.2	3.4
Public libraries	1.8	0.2
Colleges and universities	7.0	0.7
Schools	1.7	0.2
Other	2.6	2.4
Government	2.4	0.2
Industry	9.9	0.3
Special Sales	1.7	0.8
Individual Sales	18.9	32.3
By mail	18.5	18.4
Through salesmen	0.1	12.7
Convention sales	0.2	1.1
Total	100.0%	100.0%

Note: Discrepancies in totals are due to rounding.
Source: Association of American Publishers.

The key to the success of an agency plan, according to one publisher, is inventory. The publisher's salesman should regularly inventory the bookseller's shelves in order to remove old titles and replace them with the latest material. The plans make sense only if there is sizable demand for sci-tech books in the bookseller's area.

Cooperative Advertising Plans

Prentice-Hall, in the belief that general bookstores do not know how to merchandise sci-tech books, is actively trying to help them to identify potential customers, to reach them and to merchandise to them. This is being accomplished in two ways: an agency plan and a national cooperative advertising program.

In spring 1980, Prentice-Hall launched a national cooperative advertising program targeted to specific audiences as a means of making general bookstores realize the potential of the sci-tech field.

The plan began with advertisements in four trade magazines serving fields ranging from real estate to computers. Each advertisement contained Prentice-Hall titles that would appeal to the audience of a specific magazine and listed a number of bookstore accounts in various cities; the retailer shared the cost of the advertisement with the other retailers who were listed. All participants saw a rapid turnover of the three to five copies of each title that they were required to order, and most of them reordered twice before the first month was completed. In fall 1980, similar advertisements appeared in five magazines. Prentice-Hall also prepared 10 cooperative advertisements that a retailer could run in the local paper. They came with advertising mats, envelope stuffers and store display material. The company continues to operate a cooperative program.

Discounts

Most publishers of sci-tech books offer their products to retailers at short discounts averaging 20%. (Agency plan discounts generally run 30% to almost 40%.) Trade discounts sometimes may be granted, however, when a book has a consumer market. Because sci-tech books are ordered in smaller quantities than trade titles, it is more expensive for a publisher to service the account and uneconomical for it to grant a 40% discount. Since these titles are directed to a limited specific audience and, in many cases, represent a large investment by the publisher, they are generally priced higher than trade titles. Therefore, publishers feel the short discount will still yield the retailer the same dollar profit he receives on a lower-priced trade book purchased at a 40% discount.

Retail Store Sales of Medical Books

According to the AAP, retail stores accounted for 36.7% of medical book sales in 1982. General bookstores accounted for 15.0% of sales, and college bookstores and "other retailers," including medical bookstores, accounted for the remaining 21.6% of sales. (These figures are again based on the data reported by only 29 professional publishers.)

Industry spokesmen claim that most sales to bookstores are to the specialized medical bookstores; these sales are dominated by the older, more established publishers, especially those with textbook lines. Publishers of medical monographs, on the other hand, claim medical bookstores dislike stocking their publications because the unit sales are too small.

The *American Book Trade Directory—1982* lists only 113 medical bookstores. However, some of the 2718 college stores listed may carry sizable numbers of medical titles if the college has a medical school that lacks its own store. The *American Book Trade Directory—1978* listed 81 medical bookstores; thus, even allowing for undercounting in the 1978 edition, the number of medical bookstores, though small, seems to be increasing.

Ordinarily, general bookstores do not carry medical titles because of insufficient demand and because they are offered at short discounts averaging 20%. Unless a medical publisher also has a trade operation, it usually encounters difficulty in gaining entree to the general bookstore field. This situation may be changing, however. At least one general wholesaler Bookazine, is now representing an in-depth stock of medical books and giving regular medical book discounts. The demand for these books seems to be coming primarily from general bookstores located near a medical or nursing school. These outlets will order one or two copies of the two or three titles that students most often request and special order others. In addition, physicians in the area may ask the store to order certain titles.

Medical Books for the Layman

A growing interest in medical topics by the general public is certainly one of the reasons behind the 1979 decision of the W.B Saunders Co., the largest medical book publisher, to enter the trade publishing field. Saunders is publishing books on health-related topics for the lay public under two imprints—Saunders Press for hardcovers, and Saunders Paperbacks for softcover originals and reprints of Saunders Press titles. Its list includes titles such as *The Health Hypochondriac* and *Gut Reaction: How to Handle Stress and Your Stomach*.

In 1982 C.V. Mosby began publishing books for the general reader on medical topics. Titles include *Can You Prevent Cancer?* and *Women's Pharmacy: A Guide to Safe Drug Use*. The American Psychiatric Press, founded in 1981 as an affiliate of the American Psychiatric Association, planned to publish the first three titles of its new trade line in spring 1984. They include *How You Can Help: A Guide for the Families of Patients in Mental Hospitals* and *Conquer Your Phobia: A Guide Using Contextural Therapy*.

Generally, publishers who have joined the trend to producing books for laymen seem to have access to distribution channels in the trade market. Saunders' books, for example, are distributed to the trade by Holt, Reinhart and Winston, another CBS subsidiary. Publishers lacking adequate trade distribution usually find it difficult to market these books and do not seem to be entering this field.

It should be noted here that Plenum Publishing Corp. has in the last few years begun publishing a number of books dealing with scientific topics of interest to the general reader. In addition, in 1982 W.H. Freeman and Co., a subsidiary of Scientific American, established Scientific American Books to publish science books for the college and trade markets. In 1983 Little, Brown introduced the Masters of Modern Science Series, which presents ideas and writings of scientists who initiated developments and theories in modern science.

Direct Mail

The first successful promotion of a TSM title by direct mail occurred during the eighteenth century when Benjamin Franklin used this method to increase sales of his *Almanac*. Today, because retail outlets carrying TSM books are relatively few, direct mail has become a mainstay of TSM book sales and is one of the best tools available to reach the TSM reader. According to the AAP, 18.5% of the sales of sci-tech books and 18.4% of medical book sales in 1982 were to individual customers by direct mail.

Advantages

Direct mail enables a publisher to communicate directly with a potential customer without needing to compete with editorial copy or other advertising. It also permits a publisher to pinpoint his market with a fair degree of accuracy and to trace and analyze the results of his sales effort. Because TSM books are usually written by and for professionals within the same professional community, their authors are generally known to potential purchasers, a factor which makes direct mail an effective sales tool.

In addition to yielding direct sales, direct-mail selling may generate orders from other channels. This "spillover" or "echo effect" stimulates the sale of a book to customers who prefer to purchase it in a bookstore because of speed, charging privileges, and, in some cases, discounts; it may also maintain demand for a backlist title mentioned in the mailing piece. A direct-mail promotion creates requests for the book at corporate and other libraries, leading to increased library sales. One industry spokesman claims 40% of all library sales of a sci-tech title are obtained after a direct-mail campaign. One large sci-tech publisher estimates that direct mail stimulates 50% of its sci-tech sales, and others claim that a sci-tech title that sells 500 copies by direct mail will sell an additional 1200 to 1500 copies to libraries and bookstores.

Finally, in the sci-tech field, a direct-mail campaign can be employed as a catalyst for other sales activity, e.g., cooperative advertising. Often, demand for a title at the bookstore level will continue for three to four months after the launching of a direct-mail campaign if this campaign has been supported by space advertising. Thus, the overall sales activity level stimulated by a publisher's mail promotion continues to benefit bookstores and wholesalers long after the publisher's direct participation in the marketplace has come to an end.

Disadvantages

There are also disadvantages to direct-mail selling, however. Direct-mail selling is problematical because of rising costs for paper, printing and postage. In addition, since most resulting sales are of single copies, costs of fulfillment, shipping and billing are high. Nevertheless, many publishers feel that the expense of direct mail is more than offset by the high prices of the titles sold through this channel and by the already mentioned "echo effect" that results from direct-mail promotion. The effectiveness of direct mail has been somewhat blunted by shifts in scientific disciplines and "twigging," making it more difficult to pinpoint the market accurately.

Economics

A "good" return on a direct-mail promotion depends on the price of the offering. In the consumer market, where a $15 or $20 book is being sold, a good response would have to be 2.5% or better in order to realize a profit. Returns can be much lower for TSM books that sell at higher prices: a response rate of 0.6% might be acceptable in selling a $75 title.

Formulas for the ratio of direct-mail selling costs to sales differ among publishers. Many publishers believe that gross sales in a successful promotion should be two to three times direct-mail selling costs. At one company the rule of thumb is that each $1 spent on direct mail should yield $3 in orders, or a sales cost of 33%. Another believes a successful promotion can have direct-mail selling costs as high as 50% of a book's sale price, while still another believes direct-mail selling costs should be 25% of revenue.

Mail Order, Books Clubs and Continuity Series

As an alternative to direct mail sales, TSM publishers also market their books through advertisements in professional journals, book club sales and by means of continuity series.

Often an advertisement for a book contains a coupon which the customer must return in order to purchase it. Just as in the case of direct mail, this method is expensive for the publisher; sales are of single copies, necessitating high costs of billing, shipping and fulfillment. Few such ads can break even, let alone produce a profit.

Scientific and Technical Books

Book clubs are growing in importance as a means of selling sci-tech books. They extend the market for a book and may even help to keep a title alive long after its initial sale. Clubs range from those on a professional level to those on a serious hobby level. Book club readers want practical, reference and self-improvement information; the prices they are willing to pay reflect their own salary levels in their fields.

McGraw-Hill, Macmillan and Prentice-Hall are the leaders in the professional book club field. McGraw-Hill has seven sci-tech book clubs, including the Architects Book Club, Electronics and Control Engineers Book Club and the Engineers Book Society. In addition to its clubs, McGraw-Hill also operates several continuity programs on topics such as solar heating and cooling and integrated circuit technology and applications. Macmillan's eight sci-tech clubs include the Library of Computer and Information Sciences, the Library of Science and the Nature Science Book Club. Prentice-Hall's three sci-tech clubs are the Electronics Book Service, the Builders and Contractors Book Society and the Behavioral Books Institute.

In addition to the clubs owned by the above companies, there are several other sci-tech book clubs catering to both professionals and lay readers, including the Electronics Book Club, owned by TAB Books, and the Library of Human Behavior, Ltd. The Book-of-the-Month Club launched the Book-of-the-Month Club/Science, concentrating on books in the sci-tech field, in May 1981. The club capitalizes on the new interest among publishers and readers in science and is directed to professionals in the field as well as laymen. The club was expected to begin contributing to Book-of-the-Month Club profits in 1983, a remarkable performance for a new book club. In early 1983 it had 65,000 members. In addition, in late 1982 W.H. Freeman and Co., a subsidiary of Scientific American, established the Scientific American Library book club, which signed up over 21,000 members in its first three months and expected to have over 50,000 members by the beginning of 1984.

Some sci-tech publishers are more heavily involved with book club sales than others. To a large extent, the degree of involvement with book club sales depends on the type of books published. Academic Press and Elsevier North-Holland, both research publishers, sell only a few titles to book clubs, while McGraw-Hill and Van Nostrand Reinhold, professional publishers, consider book clubs an important source of sales.

Because sci-tech clubs serve a specialized market, their sales are not nearly as large as those of the general book clubs, and the volume of sales generated by a club selection varies tremendously. An alternate selection may sell 250 to 1000 copies, while a main selection may sell 1000 to 15,000 or 20,000 copies, depending on the type of book. By extending the market for a title, however, book club sales also provide the publisher with publishing economies. Since sci-tech publishing is basically a short-run industry, the unit cost of a book is lowered whenever a book club sale takes place and the club joins the publisher's print run.

The publisher's royalty is subject to negotiation in book club sales. Generally, it is 10% of the club price, shared equally between the author and publisher; however, royalties may go as low as 6%. When a title is used as a premium, the royalty is lower than when it is a club selection. Or, publishers may sell books outright to the clubs at a deep discount, e.g., 70% to 75% off list price.

Medical Books

Book clubs are of minor importance in the medical field. In 1983 IMS International Inc. launched the Medical Book Club of America, believed to be the first full-service book club for physicians only. Macmillan's Nurses Book Society serves the nursing field, and there are a few book clubs in psychology-psychiatry area, including Macmillan's Behavioral Sciences Book Club. Industry observers claim a publisher can make very little money on book club sales in the medical field. The usual royalty is 6%, shared equally with the author, and the club purchases the books from the publisher at production cost. Although a main selection may sell 20,000 to 25,000 copies in the nursing field, some titles sell considerably less. Thus, some publishers feel a club sale is beneficial only if it can bring an author's name or the company's name to the attention of the nursing community.

Another sales technique involves use of the continuity series whereby a customer agrees to receive a series of books on a particular topic at specified intervals. The customer is not required to accept a set number of books, may cancel at any time, and may return any volume he does not like. Springhouse Corp. appears to be the only medical publisher marketing its books in this manner. Currently, it is marketing three series—the Nursing Skillbook series, the Nursing Photobook series and the Nurse's Reference Library—to the 542,000 subscribers to its *Nursing '84* magazine. Titles include *Dealing with Death and Dying, Assessing Your Patients* and *Managing I.V. Therapy.*

Sales to Individuals Through Salesmen

According to the AAP, 12.7% of medical book sales in 1982 were to individuals by salesmen. (This sales technique occurs rarely in the sci-tech field.) Several medical publishers employ salesmen who call directly on doctors at their offices or at hospitals. In the past, this type of selling almost always took place on a one-to-one basis in the physician's office, but today more time is spent setting up a display in a hospital room so local physicians can examine and purchase the books. This is an expensive sales technique, but publishers find it suitable for medical books, which are generally high-priced items.

Medical meetings and conventions are also an important source of sales, especially for those publishers who do not call on individual doctors at their offices or hospitals. In many instances, a meeting or convention may afford the doctor his or her only opportunity to examine a title before purchasing it.

Libraries and Institutions

AAP figures indicate that in 1982, 13.2% of the sales of sci-tech books were to libraries and institutions, and an additional 17.7% of sales were to library jobbers, Thus, 30.9% of sci-tech book sales were to the library market, making it second in importance to sales to retail stores. In 1982, 3.4% of medical book sales were to libraries and institutions, and an additional 9.0% of sales were to library jobbers. Thus, 12.4% of medical book sales were to the library market. Direct-mail promotions are sent to libraries, but ordinarily a library makes its purchases through a library wholesaler or jobber. Few major publishers still have salesmen calling on libraries.

Libraries and institutions account for a large portion of the sales of high-priced books; thus, the shrinking of library budgets in the last few years threatens the economics of the more specialized TSM titles that depend on library sales. Libraries have been especially important in the purchase of series, advances and major treatises, although these are also purchased by laboratories and individuals. However, in the last 15 years Wiley has canceled more than 45 sci-tech series because the library market, even for these books, has shrunk due to inflation and the budget crunch.

Because of this combination of inflation and shrinking budgets, library expenditures for books are declining. Some libraries have closed, and others have no funds for acquisitions. For others, funding uncertainties have led to the spending of large sums at the close of the fiscal year.

In order to retain serial subscriptions, many research libraries are taking money away from book budgets. The National Enquiry into Scholarly Communication found that for every $1 spent on journals by large academic and research libraries in 1969, $2 was spent on books; in 1973, for every $1 spent on journals, $1 was spent on books; and in 1978, for every $1.23 spent on journals, $1 was spent on books. These figures, of course, include all types of scholarly books and journals, but it is fairly reasonable to conclude that TSM books and journals follow this pattern. The Enquiry report indicates that if these libraries are to keep their serial collections intact, the ratio of journal expenditures to book expenditures will probably rise to two-to-one or three-to-one during the 1980s.

Some industry observers also point out that growing library expenditures on computer database searching are beginning to cut into both book and journal budgets.

Textbook Market

It could be said that nearly all TSM books are used as texts because the professional who purchases them is doing so in order to increase his or her knowledge about a specific field. Most sci-tech books, however, can be used as texts or as supplementary readings by graduate students. The more advanced, higher-level titles are often used as texts by doctoral candidates. Van Nostrand Reinhold, for example, has estimated that 33% to 50% of its sci-tech titles are used at colleges in special courses and seminars, but not as basic textbooks.

In the same way, medical books with a textual orientation may be used as texts at the resident level, while a practitioner may read them simply to increase his or her knowledge. Many books, in fact, are designed to be text-references so they can enjoy dual usage.

International Sales

International markets are a major growth opportunity for TSM for TSM publishers and are becoming increasingly important to them.

Scientific and Technical Books

The world is the marketplace for a sci-tech book, especially one on an advanced level. Since the end of World War II, English has become the world's second language and the common language of science and technology. Sci-tech books from the United States are generally widely accepted abroad, regardless of nationalistic or political pressures.

Commerce Department statistics show the dollar value of U.S. exports of technical, scientific and professional books (including business, legal, medical, etc.) totaled $118.5 million in 1982, an increase of 61.6% from the $45.3 million registered in 1977. In comparison, the value of all U.S. book exports during the 1977-1982 period rose 4.1%. Thus, according to the Commerce Department, the proportion of technical, scientific and professional book exports to total book exports rose from 14.4% in 1977 to 18.5% in 1982. (See Table 3.7.)

Table 3.7 U.S. Exports of Technical, Scientific and Professional Books and Total U.S. Book Exports, 1977-1982 (Shipments Valued at $500 or More Only)[1]

Year	Technical, Scientific and Professional Books Dollars (in millions)	Units	Total Books Dollars (in millions)	Units	Technical, Scientific and Professional Books as % of Total Dollars	Units
1977	$45.3	16.2	$314.2	200.6	14.4%	8.1%
1978	49.5	16.0	370.6	226.9	13.4	7.1
1979	51.6	14.8	439.3	242.5	11.7	6.1
1980	53.9	15.8	511.6	267.0	10.5	5.9
1981	79.6	21.7	603.2	N.A.	13.2	N.A.
1982	118.5	30.6	641.3	N.A.	18.5	N.A.
% Increase: 1977-1982	161.6	88.9	104.1	N.A.[2]		

[1]Prior to August 1, 1979, shipments valued at $250 or more were included.
[2]Percent increase for the 1977-1980 period is 33.1%.
N.A. Not available.
Source: U.S. Dept. of Commerce.

The Commerce Department figures, which now exclude any shipments valued at less than $500 (thus omitting the huge volume of exports of single copies), do not correlate with industry estimates. According to these estimates, at least 20% of TSM book sales are international; combining sci-tech and medical books, this would indicate an export market of at least $140 million. Thus, the Commerce Department figures appear to be understated. Considerable additional international sales are made by the foreign subsidiaries of U.S. companies.

According to the AAP, 20.3% of sci-tech book sales were made to areas outside of the United States and Canada in 1982. The largest proportion of foreign sales, 9.9%, was to the United Kingdom and Europe, followed by 4.2% to the Asian countries (see Table 3.8). (It should be noted that only 33 professional publishers reported this information to the AAP.)

Table 3.8 Net Sales of Technical, Scientific and Medical Books, by Geographic Location, 1982

	Technical and Scientific	Medical
	(percent of total)	
United States	76.8%	86.0%
Canada	2.9	2.6
Foreign (total)	20.3	11.4
Latin America	1.5	1.5
Australia and New Zealand	1.1	1.0
Asia	4.2	2.7
United Kingdom	5.3	2.9
Africa, Near and Middle East	3.6	1.0
Continental Europe	4.6	2.4
Total	100.0	100.0

Note: Discrepancies in totals are due to rounding.
Source: Association of American Publishers.

Besides the obvious markets such as the European countries and Japan, the U.S.S.R., China and the Third World nations are also important customers for sci-tech books. The potential market for sci-tech books in China is great, given the Chinese commitment to building technological and scientific capability. Moreover, the Chinese are highly interested in sci-tech titles in English, as well as in translation rights. Nevertheless, the country's lack of a copyright law, its nonparticipation in the International Copyright Convention, and the lack of hard currency for foreign purchases are all limitations to book exports.

Medical Books

Medical titles also "travel well" abroad. According to the AAP, in 1982 11.4% of medical book sales were to areas outside of the United States and Canada. Sales to the United Kingdom and continental Europe, which were 5.3%, and sales to the Asian countries, which were 2.7%, represent the largest proportions of foreign sales (see Table 3.8). (As mentioned above, only 33 professional publishers reported this information to the AAP.) Industry spokesmen feel the AAP figure for foreign sales is extremely low and claim that about 25% to 33% of the sales of most American medical publishers are to overseas customers, with the English-speaking countries and Japan said to be the most important.

In addition to exporting their own titles, medical publishers also sell translation rights and co-publish with foreign publishers. The most advantageous situation, of course, is for a publisher to engage in both activities. Failing that, co-publishing is better for a large publisher than the sale of translation rights; since the publisher has a strong presence in the U.S. market, it can market its books successfully here. A smaller publisher may find it more advantageous to sell translation rights than to co-publish. Occasionally, a publisher will have a "hot" book on a "hot" topic that will sell in both English and the native language in a particular country. In this case, a company can sell the translation rights but can also market the English version, which will do well until the translation is released.

ECONOMICS

Figures compiled by the AAP indicate that both sci-tech books and medical books are more profitable than tradebooks. In 1982, pretax operating income of sci-tech and medical publishers was 11.0% and 7.7% of net sales, respectively, compared to 4.1% for trade book publishers (see Table 3.9). (It should be noted, however, that only 24 professional book publishers, including legal, business and other professional publishers, reported their operating data. Thus, it is likely that the figures are based on a small sample that may not be representative.)

Major differences between TSM and trade book operations occur in several areas: returns and allowances, manufacturing, royalties and "other income." In 1982, returns and allowances for sci-tech and medical books were 13.6% and 14.0% of net sales, respectively, compared to 22.5% for trade books. Returns and allowances may be a smaller portion of net sales for TSM books than for trade books because stores carrying TSM books can pinpoint their market to a great extent and, as a result, buy in more realistic quantities. It is difficult for a bookstore owner to accurately estimate his market for a potential trade best-seller, on the other hand, and he may often overbuy.

In 1982, manufacturing expenses for sci-tech and medical books were 30.7% and 30.9% of net sales, respectively, compared with 40.4% for trade books. This reflects the fact that TSM books carry much higher prices than trade books of the same page length and print run.

Table 3.9 also indicates that royalties on sci-tech and medical titles average 8.7% and 12% of net sales, respectively, while royalties on trade books average 15.9%. The difference reflects the fact that unearned advances are much more common for trade books than for TSM titles.[2]

Royalty rates offered by sci-tech publishers can range as high as 15% to 20% of sales, but 10% is average. Printed transcriptions of symposia or proceedings usually require no royalty as such, since there is no author, but a payment in the form of a royalty may be made to the sponsoring association. Average royalty for medical books is 10% of list price, sometimes rising to 11% after the first 5000 copies sold.

"Other income" was 10.7% of the net sales of trade books in 1982, compared to 5.1% and 2.7% of the net sales of sci-tech and medical books, respectively. Income from subsidiary rights, the major component of "other income," is considerably larger for trade book publishers than for TSM publishers.

TSM books are generally more profitable than trade books for several reasons. First, because TSM titles are books needed by professionals for their work, rather than titles purchased on impulse for leisure reading, the market for TSM titles is more stable than that for trade books and less affected by economic fluctuations. Second, it is relatively easy for a TSM publisher to identify and zero in on the appropriate market. Third, customers for TSM books are less price sensitive than general consumers, permitting higher margins. (Price resistance is beginning to appear, however, in the nursing and allied health areas.)

---

[2] If a trade publisher pays an advance of $15,000 against a 10% royalty, but the book sells only $100,000 worth of copies, the effective royalty is 15%; there is $5,000 in unearned advances. This is much less likely to happen in TSM publishing, since large advances are rare except for well-known authors.

Table 3.9 Operating Data of Technical and Scientific, Medical and Trade Book Publishers, 1982

	Technical and Scientific	Medical	Trade
	(percent of net sales)		
Gross sales	113.6%	114.0%	122.5%
Returns and allowances	13.6	14.0	22.5
Net sales	100.0	100.0	100.0
Cost of sales			
Manufacturing	30.7	30.9	40.4
Royalties	8.7	12.0	15.9
Total cost of sales	39.4	43.0	56.3
Gross margin on sales	60.6	57.0	43.7
Other income	5.1	2.7	10.7
Operating expense			
Editorial	8.9	8.3	6.0
Production	2.3	2.1	2.0
Marketing	19.6	18.7	16.1
Fulfillment	8.3	7.7	11.7
General and administrative	15.7	15.3	14.5
Total operating expense	54.8	52.1	50.3
Pretax income from operations	11.0%	7.7%	4.1%

Note: Discrepancies in totals are due to rounding.
Source: Association of American Publishers.

Prices

Prices of hardcover[3] TSM books are higher on the average than those of the book industry as a whole. In 1982, the average prices of scientific, technical and medical books were $44.44, $40.65 and $38.88, respectively,

---

[3]Trade paperback sci-tech and medical titles are not a significant factor in the market.

compared to an industrywide average of $30.34. Prices of sci-tech books have risen steadily since 1970. Thus prices of science titles rose from $14.95 in 1970 to $44.44 in 1982, a 197.3% increase, and prices of technical titles rose 172.6% from $14.91 in 1970 to $40.65 in 1982. Prices of medical titles, on the other hand, declined during the early 1970s but have risen steadily since 1974. The average price of a medical book dropped from $18.05 in 1970 to $15.92 in 1973 and then rose to $38.88 in 1982, a 115.4% increase over the entire period. Prices of hardcover books as a whole rose 162.3%—less than sci-tech but more than medical titles—during this period.

The combined prices of hardcover sci-tech titles increased at a faster pace during the 1970s and early 1980s than the prices of items in the Consumer Price Index, which rose 148.6% from 1970 to 1982. Prices of hardcover and medical books, on the other hand, rose at a slower pace during this period than the prices of items in the Index.

The higher prices of sci-tech and medical books, relative to other titles, reflect not only buyers' willingness to pay the prices but also higher publication costs. Although composition costs per page may be identical for a trade book and a TSM book, the TSM book market is smaller and more limited. Thus, a publisher must recover plant costs from a relative handful of people and must price its books accordingly.

Many TSM books require high-quality, expensive production. Good-quality paper must be used for reproductive purposes. The use of highly detailed illustrations (often in color) and diagrams greatly increases plant costs. The use of draftsmen to produce the diagrams raises costs, and the plates themselves are expensive. In addition, tables, formulas and other technical details commonly included in these books must be carefully checked, which is a costly process.

Cost and Revenue Models

The size of a first printing depends on several factors, including the reputation of the book's author, the estimated size of the market for the book and the experience of the publisher.

Sci-tech publishing tends to be short-run because of the specificity of its subject matter, which results in some disciplines being limited to relatively few people. The size of a print run can vary widely, however. First runs can range from 300 copies to 25,000 copies, but the great majority are under 5000 copies. Ordinarily, the printing for a research publication intended for scientific researchers or a highly specialized monograph will range from 1000 to 3000 copies; some printings are as low as several hundred. (In the case of these short-run titles, reprints are rarely feasible, so the publisher must price the book high enough to make a profit by selling most or all of the first printing. Library and institutional sales are the bulwark of this sort of publishing, and plant costs can be kept low by typewriter composition, or by having authors submit camera-ready pages.) A professional publication, directed to those involved in a specific field, will have a run of 2000 to 5000 copies; if it is a solid title, the run may be 7500 to 8500 copies or more.

Medical publishing also tends to be short-run, though perhaps less so than sci-tech publishing. The size of a first printing may range from a low of 1500 copies for an esoteric monograph to more than 20,000 copies for a book on anatomy. It should be kept in mind that the monograph with a run of 1500 copies may have better penetration of its limited market than the title with a run in the tens of thousands. The average medical book has a run of 2500 to 5000 copies, however. Short print runs, together with high plant costs, result in high prices for TSM titles. The use of color in medical books is also increasingly expensive. As a result, some publishers discourage the use of color; if an author insists upon its use, he or she must find funding to cover the extra costs.

PAPERBACKS, BACKLIST AND REVISIONS

Paperbacks

Some paperback publishing occurs in the TSM field. There is no difference in plant or printing costs between a paperback and a hardcover original, however; the only difference between the two, in fact, is the binding. Thus, publishing an original title in paperback should not be viewed as a means of significantly lowering costs. If a paperback title is a reprint, however, plant costs were already incurred with the hardcover edition. Therefore, after the investment has been recovered, a title may be sometimes reprinted and priced as low as possible. For example, one publisher produced an 835-page book for $45 and later marketed a softcover edition for $22.50. Occasionally, when a title has a potential use as a supplementary text, a publisher will print a paperback edition simultaneously with the hardcover title.

Paperback publishing in the medical field is used most often for nursing titles, which are predominantly textbooks. The market for medical books is primarily a hardcover market. When a physician purchases a reference book, he or she wants it to be durable and long-lasting, and paperbound books have a bad connotation. However, some medical books are being produced with sturdy softcover or limp bindings, using Lexan, Kivar or other synthetic materials.

Backlist

Scientific and Technical Books

As is true of other sectors of the publishing industry, backlist sales are quite important to the sci-tech publisher. A typical sci-tech title may sell 2000 copies in its first two or three years and then sales will taper off; total sales in the book's five to seven years of life may eventually reach 2500 copies. Probably over 50% of these sales will take place after the first year of publication (i.e., when the book is a backlist title). Many publishers estimate that 60% to 70% of their sci-tech sales are from their backlists.

The first printing of a research book is normally expected to last 18 to 24 months. This may be its lifetime sale, especially if it is a monograph or a title funded by a research grant. Elsevier, primarily a publisher of research titles, has found that because of the topicality of its material, 50% of its sales take place in the first year after publication, and 80% to 90% occur in the first two years. The life of the average professional book, on the other hand, is about five years. If there are many new developments in its field, however, a title will become obsolete quickly; if the field remains stable, it will sell well for a long period of time, and some books may remain on a backlist for 10 to 15 years. Therefore, it is difficult to predict the average sale of a sci-tech title over its life; this depends on the subject matter and the market.

Medical Books

The life of a medical book and, therefore, the importance of backlist sales, can vary widely. Year Book, for example, finds that once a yearbook is established in a field, the company is able to estimate the number of copies to be sold each year. Each book has only one press run; the life of each book is no more than a year, and backlist sales are practically nonexistent. Raven Press finds that its titles age quickly, and most sales take place within the first two years after publication. Little, Brown, on the other hand, still has the first medical book it published in 1954 in print in the same edition. Generally some 50% to 60% of medical book sales are from the backlist, but this proportion will vary with the maturity of the company's list and the types of books published.

Some industry observers point out that because of the increasing number of publishers and books published in the last few years, backlist sales have decreased in importance, and the average life of a clinical title has dropped from four years to two years.

Reprints or Revisions

The period within which a book is revised or a new edition is printed usually depends on the subject matter and on what other books on the same subject have been published in the interim. It is costly to revise a book. Sometimes a title may need revision within a year or two, but this is too expensive an undertaking until all the initial costs have been recovered. A publisher with a large backlist, on the other hand, may concentrate on revising books (and revise them frequently), thus taking fewer risks than with the publication of new titles.

Ordinarily, a revision or new edition of a book is published every four to six years, if a market for it still exists; however, one publisher says books on high technology currently have a useful life of three years. Some titles may go for 10 years or more without revision, however. The amount of new material contained in a revision varies depending on the subject matter and competition. One medical publisher attempts to present 25% new material in its revised editions, but sometimes competitive factors will force revision with less.

When a book is revised, it is usually considered to be a new title, and the publishing economies are those of a new book. There is a great deal of new editorial matter, new publicity, new rights sales, etc. The publisher now has a fairly accurate idea of the size of its market and has a more receptive and optimistic attitude toward pricing the title because it has been a proven success. Issuing a new edition or revision endows a book with the characteristics of a classic, and this momentum picks up new customers. In addition, people who already own the book frequently purchase each new edition. Sometimes, however, they may "leapfrog" one revision by postponing their purchase until the next edition. In a growing market it is difficult to tell the amount of "leapfrogging" that is taking place because more copies of the newest edition will be sold as a result of the increase in market size since the publication of the original edition.

Thor Power Tool Case

Despite the fact that backlist sales are extremely important in the publishing industry, the 1979 Supreme Court decision in *Thor Power Tool Co. v. the Commissioner of Internal Revenue* has forced all publishers to reconsider the economics of backlist sales. This decision upheld an Internal Revenue Service (IRS) ruling against Thor Power Tool Co. that depreciation on warehoused goods could not be written off unless they were sold at reduced cost or destroyed. Thus, it would not be possible for a publisher to reduce the value of an overstocked title for tax purposes unless the books were sold at reduced cost or physically destroyed.

The practice of writing down the value of inventory is especially common among TSM publishers. These titles do not appeal to remainder store customers and, often, the smaller publishers have inventories too small for a remainder house to bother to handle. Changing markets, new scientific or technological developments or simply the publication of a new book on the identical subject can make a backlist title obsolete. Good accounting practice states that the book value of the inventory should be reduced to less than cost, if that represents its present market value. The amount by which the asset value of inventories is lowered on the balance sheet becomes an expense on the income statement and results in reduced income taxes.

Though they may sell slowly, backlist titles often continue to sell for several years. Their sales gradually reduce inventory, help to build a strong backlist, and yield small profits, which, in turn, help the publisher to bring out new titles. The 1979 ruling, if allowed to stand, forces publishers, especially the smaller ones, to destroy their inventories of slow sellers in order to realize the tax benefits of inventory writedowns.

In the future, if sales of a book do not meet expectations one or two years after publication, existing copies may be destroyed and the book permitted to go out of print. Thus, one outcome of the *Thor* ruling could be smaller print runs, which will raise unit costs and prices and increase out-of-stock conditions. Another could be the decision not to publish books of marginal commercial appeal, such as scholarly works.

Though the *Thor* ruling has provoked angry criticism from the publishing industry, it may have some salutory effects as well, such as alerting publishers to pay sharper attention to the hidden costs of keeping titles in print (e.g., warehouse space and the cost of money), more realistic cost accounting, and a determination to write off all nonrecurring publication costs (plant, editorial and promotion) in the year of publication.

According to an ALA publication from December 1983, evidence of the effect on publishers' backlists is mixed. Some companies have felt the effects, but others have been in compliance with the inventory methods upheld in the Thor decision for years. Several legislative remedies have been proposed in recent years. In November 1983 Sen. Daniel Moynihan (D-NY) introduced a bill proposing that if a publishing house, based on its most recent five-year experience, could demonstrate that a portion of its inventory of books and other published material will eventually be sold below cost, it could write down that portion to its net realizable value. "Books or other published material" is defined to include "books, maps, sheet music, monographs, periodicals and similar printed works."

NONPROFIT PUBLISHERS

Publishing operations in a nonprofit organization differ in many ways from those of a commercial publisher. Nonprofit publishers tend to publish on a smaller scale, with fewer titles, shorter print runs and lower markups. As a result, they have less clout when shopping for paper and printing and less capital available for taking risks. Staffs are usually smaller, with lower salaries, a factor that leads to high turnover and makes these organizations an ideal training ground for large professional publishers.

On the other hand, governmental assistance is often available to a nonprofit publisher in the form of grants, favorable postage rates or a tax-exempt status. The association's membership becomes its primary customer; often when members join a professional society, they identify their fields of interest so that mailings describing books in their specialty can be directed to them. Nonprofit publishers can also exchange information without fear of charges of collusion, and because their staffs are smaller and generally more dedicated, they can assume more responsibilities. Finally, because they are not concerned with showing a profit, nonprofit publishers are more likely to publish books which, though important to the profession, may not be successful commercially.

Nonprofit Associations as Book Publishers

Nonprofit publishers are more important in the journal field than in the book field. However, the Institute of Electrical and Electronics Engineers (IEEE) and the American Chemical Society are among those organizations that have some type of book publishing program.

American Chemical Society

The American Chemical Society prints a small number of monographs annually, in addition to about 40 book titles, the majority of which are proceedings and symposia of the 128,000-member organization. Usually the society prints about 1500 copies in a first print run, and the book is not reprinted. Titles are sold by direct mail to members and others in the chemistry field, to libraries and to sci-tech bookstores. This nonprofit publisher's financial goal is to do slightly better than breaking even; in 1980 its estimated book sales were about $1.5 million. In 1982 book sales totaled $1.9 million, of which 30% were to foreign countries.

Institute of Electrical and Electronics Engineers (IEEE)

Although the IEEE is primarily a publisher of journals, its IEEE Press publishes reprint volumes containing selected articles drawn mostly, but not exclusively, from IEEE literature. It publishes several of these books a year in addition to conference proceedings and standards books and, occasionally, it publishes an original work. Recently IEEE Press began an expansion program; it is planning to publish 20 to 30 books annually, including original titles.

The organization tries to run its book publishing operations in a similar manner to those of a commercial publisher. It has a well-defined market represented by its membership of 230,000, which is appealing to authors and guest editors. IEEE has 84 books now in print. Members receive a discount of 20% to 40% off list price. Usually a first printing is 3000 to 5000 copies. Camera-ready copy is used almost exclusively, as IEEE books can be photoreproduced from its journals.

In 1980 sales of the IEEE Press alone were about $500,000; proceedings and standards accounted for an additional $1 million to $1.5 million. Thus, total IEEE sales of books were about $1.5 million to $2 million.

ENCYCLOPEDIAS AND HANDBOOKS

Encyclopedias

Scientific and technical encyclopedias are intended for professionals rather than for college students; these people do not want to take a course in a subject, but are seeking a reference book that will furnish the information they desire in a few pages.

Encyclopedias are more profitable than other sci-tech books. Because they are usually purchased on a subscription basis, a publisher is better able to estimate their potential sales and adjust print runs accordingly. They are targeted to a specific audience and are considered basic work tools, factors which result in an inelastic market and ease in pricing. In addition, a publisher is not locked into a specific price on the entire series; he can set a price on the first few volumes of a multivolume encyclopedia and then raise it, if necessary, on the next few volumes. Because of their high prices, encyclopedias are primarily purchased by libraries and institutions and, therefore, have a lower return factor than other sci-tech titles. Finally, one encyclopedia is ordinarily not competitive with another.

Publishing economics for encyclopedias are similar to those for other sci-tech titles, except for the necessary high investment. Because of high plant costs, salaries and overhead, it may cost upwards of $70 per page to develop an encyclopedia, and it is not unusual for a multivolume encyclopedia to incur an upfront investment of $1.5 million to $2 million or more. Revisions are also costly; plant costs for the sixth edition of the *Van Nostrand Scientific Encyclopedia*, for example, were approximately $500,000.

It should be noted that the market for an encyclopedia may be larger than that for a sci-tech book. Although the length of a print run varies with the subject, it usually is between 6000 to 12,000 copies. Annual sales may total 4000 to 8000 sets; however, some purchasers may buy only certain volumes because they are interested in specific articles.

The frequency of revision for an encyclopedia depends on the subject matter. Generally, however, an encyclopedia is revised every six to 10 years, because the publisher needs time to recoup its investment on each edition before starting over. The proportion of new material in a revision varies and may range from 20% to 65%. Libraries and other institutions or individuals often continue to buy single volumes or complete sets of an older edition even after a new edition is in print. They may prefer the format of the earlier edition, or it may contain articles that have become "classics" in the literature of the field.

Normally, encyclopedias are sold by direct mail. Although sales by distribution channel may vary from one encyclopedia to another, libraries and institutions usually account for the majority of sales. While libraries can do without many acquisitions during this time of shrinking budgets and high prices, encyclopedias—especially for a population highly concerned with technology—are mandatory.

Wiley, McGraw-Hill and Van Nostrand Reinhold are the leaders in the sci-tech encyclopedia area. Wiley publishes three multivolume encyclopedias: the *Encyclopedia of Polymer Science and Technology,* the 26-volume *Encyclopedia of Chemical Technology* (ed. Kirk-Othmer), and the *Encyclopedia of Statistical Sciences.* In early 1984 it published the *Encyclopedia of Psychology.* McGraw-Hill publishes several encyclopedias, of which the most important is *The Encyclopedia of Science and Technology*. Van Nostrand Reinhold publishes 14 encyclopedias, including the two-volume, 3000-page *Van Nostrand Scientific Encyclopedia*, which claims to be America's most widely used scientific encyclopedia. The company's other encyclopedias include *Encyclopedia of Minerals* and *Encyclopedia of Computer Science*.

Handbooks

A handbook differs from an encyclopedia in that it focuses on a subject from various points of view and is organized by topics. It definitively covers its subject and is often considered the Bible of its specific discipline. Individuals tend to purchase handbooks because they are considered essential work tools and are less expensive than encyclopedias. For this reason, sales of handbooks are often higher than encyclopedia sales. Wiley, McGraw-Hill and Van Nostrand Reinhold are leading publishers of sci-tech handbooks.

OUTLOOK

Scientific and Technical Books

Sales of sci-tech books are expected to continue to be strong during the next five years. Scientific research probably will continue to enjoy reasonable levels of public and private financial support in amounts that will keep pace with inflation, because of the support of the military-industrial establishment plus that of the large professional societies. However, any cuts in library or research funding will have an adverse effect on sales.

Enrollments in college engineering courses are strong, and there is a continuing need for the most current information in the field. Graduate enrollments in the sciences will benefit from decreased interest in humanistic studies and will remain stable, if not increasing. A growing number of mid-career changes and the trend to lifelong learning will also help to assure the growth of sci-tech publishing. The overseas market may well be the fastest-growing market for sci-tech books despite unstable political environments and fluctuating currencies.

Books on engineering, robotics, automation, computer sciences, environmental science and energy should have sizable markets between now and the late 1980s. However, publishers must stay alert to the creation of new disciplines or subdisciplines so their publishing programs will remain current.

Competition will be stronger in the next five years. In the past, a new title could live without competition for some time, but now a similar title may appear in the marketplace within months. Publishers must remember that books are merely a means of communication, and that they must be prepared for increased competition from other media forms, such as online databases. Finally, there will be competition from European publishers who are increasingly establishing American branches, seeking American authors, printing their books in English and publishing books in this country.

It is likely that by 1986, sales of sci-tech books will reach $580 million, a 34.4% increase over 1982; by 1989 sales are expected to total $700 million, a 62.4% increase over 1982. (See Table 3.1 for 1982 sci-tech sales figures.)

Medical Books

Sales of medical books are expected to continue to be strong during the next five years. Although the number of doctors, dentists and other professionals in the health fields is continuing to increase, it should be kept in mind, according to industry experts, that many physicians rarely purchase books after completing medical school; they instead rely on detail men (sales reps for pharmaceutical companies) and medical journals in order to stay up-to-date. Requirements for continuing medical education may help book sales; however, there are other means of obtaining the necessary credits.

Increasing specialization will provide a base for future growth. More books on more subjects will be published, but fewer units of each will be sold, resulting in rising costs because of shorter runs. Changing methods of diagnosis, new medical technology (such as the use of ultrasound techniques) and new treatments for diseases (such as diabetes and asthma) will also result in a need for books which can keep clinicians apprised of new developments.

Because of the proliferation of medical publishing houses in recent years, the field has become quite competitive. Many publishers feel a shakeout of weak companies will occur during the 1980s, with the exact timing depending on the economic situation. The larger publishers with high-quality products and extensive marketing resources will survive. Relatively small publishers or small medical divisions of general publishers may go under, but there will always be room for the small publisher of quality books. Smaller publishers may be forced to specialize or to depend on symposia proceedings.

It is likely that by 1986 medical book sales will have reached $360 million, a 34.1% increase over 1982; by 1989 sales will probably total $425 million, 58.3% above the 1982 figure. (See Table 3.1 for 1982 medical book sales figures.)

4

Magazines and Journals

Revenue from magazine and journal publishing in the technical, scientific and medical (TSM) field totaled an estimated $893 million in 1982.

DIFFERENCES BETWEEN MAGAZINES AND JOURNALS

Although librarians have often encountered difficulty over the years in defining the terms "magazine" and "journal," and some people involved in TSM publishing use the two terms interchangeably, there are actually distinct differences between them. Fritz Machlup and Kenneth Leeson and associates have stated that "...magazines are written chiefly for the general reader, whereas journals are for readers specialized in a particular discipline or interested in intellectually sophisticated treatments of a variety of subjects."[1] This broad distinction ignores the fact that the TSM field contains both magazines and journals which are intended for readers "in a particular discipline."

According to the Association of American Publishers (AAP), a primary journal contains works of research and is aimed at a professional audience (technical, scientific, medical, or scholarly). It is generally a monthly in which articles appear for the first time and are subject to peer review by a group of professionals.

---

[1] Machlup, Fritz, Leeson, Kenneth et al., *Information Through the Printed Word, The Dissemination of Scholarly Scientific and Intellectual Knowledge, Volume 2: Journals,* Praeger Publishers, 1978.

Scientific and Technical Magazines and Journals

Some members of scientific and technical (sci-tech) fields point out that a journal should contribute something to the knowledge of a profession. It is a scholarly publication devoted to the first announcement of research or to original works written by the individuals who conducted the research. It publishes peer-reviewed material rather than contributed material and is concerned with a specific field rather than with a general area. Its frequency is usually quarterly to bimonthly, and it may be affiliated with a professional association.

A journal attracts a smaller audience than a magazine; its purpose is not to have popular appeal, and some expertise in a field may be necessary in order to read it. Editors of journals are often noted researchers or professionals. In addition, a journal usually does not pay for its material; in fact, in many instances an author may be charged a fee for the publication of his work. Generally, a journal is supported by subscription rather than advertising revenue. The concept of peer review, it should be noted, is basic to the definition of a journal. Peer review is the review of a submitted article by one or more individuals in the field about which the article is written; their comments and recommendations for changes are passed on to the authors. Thus, peer review is a means of deciding whether an article submitted to a journal is scientifically sound and worth publishing.

Magazines, on the other hand, provide an overview of a subject and contain news and applications of research often written by members of the publication's staff. The articles tend to be reviews rather than original data. In most cases there is no peer review, and the publication pays for material submitted by outside contributors. Moreover, a magazine is usually supported by advertising revenue.

Medical Magazines and Journals

In the medical publishing field, the confusion of terms persists. Some publishers do not really differentiate between a journal and a magazine and call most periodicals dealing with clinical issues "journals," while other publications—such as *Medical Economics*, which deals with the financial aspects of running a practice—are considered "magazines."

Another distinction will be used throughout this chapter, however. It involves two basic differences between journals and magazines in the medical field: peer review and subscription revenue. As in the sci-tech area, articles in a medical journal are subject to peer review and their contents are devoted to reports of research, generally written by the person who conducted the research. Another parallel with journals in the sci-tech field is that a medical journal ordinarily does not pay for its material, and, in some instances, may charge an author a fee for the publication of his work. Readers are always required to pay for a medical journal, although this fee may be included in their dues if the publication is the official journal of an association. Unlike a sci-tech journal, however, a medical journal may carry a fair amount of advertising. Advertisements, usually for clinical drugs, are generally placed at the front and back of an issue; there may also be a "well" of eight to 12 advertising pages between articles or at the beginning of a new section.

A medical magazine, on the other hand, is a health-care publication that is not academic or research-directed in nature. It is a periodical published independently for profit that provides physicians and other health professionals with information related to their profession, and it usually pays its writers for their editorial contributions. In most cases a magazine does not have peer review and is a controlled circulation publication; that is, its readers do not pay to receive it. It is supported entirely or primarily by advertising, and its advertisements may be interspersed throughout its editorial pages.

SIZE AND STRUCTURE OF THE MARKET

Statistics on the size of the TSM market for magazines and journals are woefully inadequate. There seem to be no annual compilations of the number of TSM magazines and journals or of their total circulation and advertising revenue.

Number of Magazines and Journals

TSM magazines and journals can be divided into two categories, sci-tech and medical. Because of the differences in terminology discussed above, we shall continue to treat sci-tech and medical magazines and journals as separate categories in this section.

Scientific and Technical Magazines

Although there are many magazines serving the sci-tech fields, the great majority of them are directed to marketing and management personnel, rather than to scientific and technical professionals. Because these periodicals tend to carry more news and marketing data than reports of scientific and technical developments, this study will consider them business or trade periodicals rather than sci-tech publications. Examples of this type of periodical are *Engineering News Record, Oil & Gas Journal,* and *Chemical Week.*

In the last few years there also has been increased interest in the publication of scientific magazines for the lay reader. At present there are four major magazines in this category—*Scientific American, Science 84, Discover* and *Science Digest.* Although *Scientific American,* the oldest of the four publications, was never intended for the casual reader and while its circulation of about 708,000 in the United States and abroad is primarily composed of scientists and engineers, *Standard Rate and Data*—the final arbiter in these matters—classifies it as a consumer magazine. *Science 84,* introduced in 1979 as a bimonthly by the American Association for the Advancement of Science (AAAS), began publishing 10 times a year in November 1980 and has a circulation of 727,000. The publication has an inside pipeline to the scientific community because of its ties to the AAAS. This organization, on the other hand, has its own 100-year-old *Science* journal, intended for the professional scientist.

Time Inc. began publishing *Discover,* a monthly with circulation of 878,000, in October 1980. Its venture into this field was prompted by the high newsstand sales achieved by *Time* magazine whenever its cover story would deal with a subject related to science, medicine or behavior. In October 1980, the Hearst Corp. began publishing *Science Digest* monthly in an 8½-inch by 11-inch page size; the old *Science Digest* had been digest-sized, and was published bimonthly. *Science Digest* currently has a circulation of 530,000.

There are relatively few magazines directed to professionals in the sci-tech field. The actual number, in fact, is probably less than 100. The important magazines in this sector are those published by three professional associations—Institute of Electrical and Electronics Engineers (IEEE), American Chemical Society and American Institute of Physics—and include *IEEE Spectrum, Chemical and Engineering News* and *Physics Today.*

Scientific and Technical Journals

Estimates of the number of sci-tech journals currently published in the United States range from a low of 1000 to a peak figure of 18,000 to 20,000. In 1980 F.W. Faxon Co., a library subscription agent for magazines and journals, listed 3106 entries in its database for scientific periodicals and an additional 2873 entries for publications concerned with technology, a total of 5979 entries. Although these figures included magazines, microfiche and newspapers in addition to journals, and were for all countries of origin, they provide an indication that fewer than 6000 sci-tech journals are published in the United States today.

Further, in 1975, Donald King counted 4175 sci-tech journals published in the United States, of which 2253 were scholarly journals primarily devoted to the reporting of research results, and 1922 were "other" sci-tech journals.[2] It is likely, then, that there are currently between 4000 and 5000 sci-tech journals published in the United States.

Medical Magazines and Journals

The confusion in terminology between magazines and journals that exists in the medical field is one factor that makes it extremely difficult, if not impossible, to obtain reliable separate estimates of the number of medical magazines and journals.

In 1980 one industry expert estimated that there were about 150 to 160 major medical-surgical magazines and journals directed to physicians engaged in primary patient care. In addition, about 50 major publications dealt with medical-related areas, such as hematology, pathology, etc., and another 100 major magazines served the nursing, hospital and dental fields, for a total of 300 major publications. The same expert pointed out that the total of all medical journals and magazines, including county and state medical journals, probably approached 4000. However, in 1980 F.W. Faxon's database listed 2210 entries for medical publications, regardless of the country of origin and including microfiche and newspapers in addition to journals and magazines.

The April 24, 1983, issue of Standard Rate and Data Service's *Business Publication Rates and Data* lists 407 magazines and journals in the medical-surgical group; 58, in the nursing and health category; 41, in the dental group; 15, in the health care classification; and 19, in the hospital administration category, for a total of 540 medical magazines and journals. It is likely that many journals and magazines are not included in this tabulation because they have not applied for a listing in SRDS or they are unable to meet the requirements for listing, which are related to the amount of national advertising carried in each issue. In addition, state and local society journal groups were excluded from the above tabulation.

Ulrich's International Periodicals Directory 1982, on the other hand, lists 1750 publications in its medical and related health-care categories; however, this figure includes newsletters, local county bulletins and college alumni bulletins.

It is likely, however, that the number of U.S.-published medical

---

[2]King, Donald W. et al., *Statistical Indicators of Scientific and Technical Communication (1960-1980)*, King Research Inc. for the NSF, 1976-1977.

magazines and journals—excluding local, county and state publications—is between 1200 and 3000.

Size of the Market

Whereas the size of the magazine industry is generally measured in terms of advertising revenue only, many journals, especially those in the sci-tech category and in small medical specialties, have little or no advertising revenue. Therefore, in order to measure the size of the TSM magazine and journal industry, this report will include both advertising and subscription revenue of magazines and journals.

Subscription Revenue

Machlup and Leeson estimate that revenue from subscriptions for all scholarly and scientific journals, including medical journals, published in the United States in 1973 totaled $203 million. Allowing for inflation and an increase in the number of journals, revenue from subscriptions to TSM journals probably totaled about $600 million in 1982, with medical journals accounting for about $200 million and sci-tech publications for the remaining $400 million. Since the majority of medical magazines have controlled circulation, subscription revenue from medical magazines is practically nil. Subscription revenue from the less than 100 sci-tech magazines directed to sci-tech professionals is estimated at $12 to $18 million. Thus, total subscription revenue from TSM magazines and journals was probably about $618 million in 1982.

Advertising Revenue

Advertising revenue of sci-tech journals and magazines is small, probably amounting to about $25 million, evenly divided between the scientific and technical categories. Advertising revenue of medical magazines and journals, on the other hand, totals about $250 million, 10 times the amount generated by sci-tech journals and magazines. Thus, in 1982, advertising revenue from TSM magazines and journals is estimated to have totaled about $275 million. These estimates are summarized in Table 4.1.

Leading Magazines

The 25 leading TSM magazines in 1982, in terms of total revenue from advertising and subscriptions, are listed in Table 4.2. These 25 publications

Table 4.1 Sci-Tech and Medical Magazines and Journals, by Subscription and Advertising Revenue, 1982 (in millions)

	Subscription Revenue	Subscription Revenue as % of Total	Advertising Revenue	Advertising Revenue as % of Total	Total Revenue
Magazines					
Sci-tech	$18	59.0%	$12.5	41.0%	$30.5
Medical	0	0	165.0	100.0	165.0
Subtotal	$18	9.2	$177.5	90.8	$195.5
Journals					
Sci-tech	$400	97.0%	$12.5	3.0	$412.5
Medical	200	70.2	85.0	29.8	285.0
Subtotal	$600	86.0	$ 97.5	14.0	$697.2
Total	$618	69.2	$275	30.8%	$893

Source: Knowledge Industry Publications, Inc.

accounted for total revenues of $233.9 million, or 26.2% of estimated total industry revenue; 82.1% of their revenue came from advertising, while subscription revenue accounted for the remaining 17.9%.

Only six of the 25 listed magazines and journals are concerned with scientific and technical subjects; the remaining 19 publications are directed to physicians and other health professionals. In addition, only four of these publications—*Science, New England Journal of Medicine, Journal of the American Medical Association* and *Annals of Internal Medicine*—are considered journals under the definition employed in this study; the remaining periodicals are classified as magazines.

Leading Publishers

The 15 leading U.S. publishers of TSM magazines and journals in terms of total 1980 revenue (advertising and subscription revenue) are listed in Table 4.3. Revenue of these 15 companies totaled an estimated $203.3 million in 1980, or 26.9% of total estimated TSM revenue from journals and magazines. It should be noted, however, that several large journal publishers, such as Elsevier North-Holland and Pergamon Press, are not included in this list because they are subsidiaries of European corporations.

Ten of the 15 leading publishers were publishers of journals rather than magazines; thus, it cannot be said that journal publishing is small business. In addition, six of the 15 leading publishers, or 40%, were not-for-profit

Table 4.2 Total Estimated Revenue From Advertising and Subscriptions of 25 Leading Technical, Scientific and Medical Magazines and Journals, 1982 (revenues in thousands)

Magazine	Estimated Advertising Revenue	Estimated Subscription Revenue	Estimated Total Revenue	Estimated 1982 Average Circulation
New England Journal of Medicine	$9,900	$9,337	$19,237	204,313
Medical Economics	18,189	982	19,171	182,693
Machine Design	16,500	0	16,500	165,416
Science	6,725	7,725	14,451	157,658
Nursing '82	6,841	7,244	14,085	545,712
Journal of the American Medical Association	12,289	1,043	13,332	290,836
Plant Engineering	12,714	0	12,714	100,437
Chemical Engineering	11,133	1,531	12,664	69,970
American Journal of Nursing	3,995	4,835	8,829	345,329
RN Magazine	3,672	4,886	8,558	374,830
Diversion	8,467	0	8,467	176,215
Patient Care	7,644	0	7,644	108,823
Consultant	7,076	0	7,076	120,566
Annals of Internal Medicine	3,643	3,220	6,863	91,959
Hospital Practice	6,739	0	6,739	195,729
Emergency Medicine	6,500	0	6,500	123,737
American Medical News	6,407	26	6,433	329,352
MD Magazine	6,240	0	6,240	154,442
American Family Physician	6,048	0	6,048	120,273
Medical World News	5,866	160	6,026	115,917
Postgraduate Medicine	5,665	0	5,665	137,514
Modern Medicine	5,638	0	5,638	119,699
Power	4,606	652	5,258	54,900
Electronic Products	4,915	0	4,915	116,516
Petroleum Engineer International	4,716	130	4,845	30,066
Total	$192,128	$41,771	$233,898	$4,432,902

Source: Folio: The Magazine for Magazine Management, The Folio: 400, Folio Magazine Publishing Corp., October 1983.

associations, an indicator that nonprofit publishing is not necessarily synonymous with small business. Finally, although few of the leading TSM magazines or journals deal with sci-tech subjects, five of the leading publishers were producers of sci-tech journals.

Table 4.3 Estimated Revenue of 15 Leading Publishers of Technical, Scientific and Medical Magazines and Journals, 1980 (in millions)

Rank	Publisher	Estimated Revenue[1]
1	Medical Economics	$27.0
2	Academic Press (including Grune & Stratton)	20.0
3	American Medical Association	16.5
4	American Institute of Physics	16.0[2]
5	McGraw-Hill Publications Co.	15.0
6	American Chemical Society	13.5
6	Harcourt Brace Jovanovich	13.5
7	Springhouse Corp.[3]	12.0
8	The C.V. Mosby Co.	11.0
8	The Williams & Wilkins Co.	11.0
9	New England Journal of Medicine	10.5
9	Plenum Publishing Corp.	10.5
10	American Journal of Nursing Co.	10.0
11	Harper & Row, Publishers, Inc.	8.8
12	The Institute of Electrical and Electronics Engineers, Inc.	8.0
	Total	$203.3
	Estimated industry revenue	$755.0
	15 leading companies as percent of total	26.9%

Note: In 1980 W.B. Saunders Co. published 14 Clinics and three journals with an estimated combined revenue of $10 million; however, the Clinics were considered neither magazines nor journals.
[1]Figures represent advertising and circulation revenue from each publisher's magazines and journals in the technical, scientific and medical categories. In some instances, estimates also include page charges.
[2]Figure includes both American Institute of Physics (AIP) revenue and revenue for the account of AIP member societies for publishing activities carried on for them by the AIP. Figure also includes an estimated $5 million in voluntary page charges.
[3]Formerly Intermed Communications.
Sources: Company annual reports; Knowledge Industry Publications, Inc. estimates.

SCIENTIFIC AND TECHNICAL MAGAZINES

Most periodicals serving the sci-tech sector are journals rather than magazines. The important magazines in this field, however, are those published by three not-for-profit associations—The Institute of Electrical and Electronics Engineers (IEEE), the American Chemical Society (ACS) and the American Institute of Physics (AIP).

IEEE publishes *IEEE Spectrum* plus 11 other magazines, including *Design & Test of Computers Magazine*, which will be launched in 1984. *IEEE Spectrum* is distributed to all Institute members and is one of the benefits members receive in exchange for their dues. An IEEE member also has the option of joining one or more of its 35 member societies and councils, and three of its magazines are official society publications distributed automatically to their members.

IEEE Spectrum, which in 1983 had a circulation of 230,000, had estimated revenue of $4.8 million in 1982, of which $3.2 million was derived from advertising. (In 1982, that magazine's circulation was 214,000.) In addition to product and instrumentation advertising, the magazine carries institutional and employment advertising. In 1980 it introduced *IEEE Spectrum Select* (now known as the "Consumer Edition"), a demographic edition that offers the advertiser 210,000 upscale readers in the United States and Canada and accepts advertising for selected consumer products and services, such as automobiles, cameras and travel.

ACS publishes *Chemical & Engineering News*, which is sent automatically to all 131,000 members of the Society; *Folio* magazine estimated the magazine's 1982 revenues at $7.8 million, of which $5.4 million was derived from advertising. It is a newsweekly designed to keep its readers informed of all the news of the chemical world (including marketing and management news) as it relates to the universe at large.

The AIP publishes *Physics Today*, which goes automatically to all its members and has a circulation of 75,000. The magazine tries to keep physicists abreast of all disciplines. The main support of *Physics Today* is advertising revenue, which totals about $1.4 million annually.

MEDICAL MAGAZINES

Estimates of the number of publications that the average general practitioner receives each month range from 60 to 110 and include national, regional and local magazines and journals, plus magazines such as *Medical Economics* and *Diversion* that are devoted to the economics of a practice and activities available to those in high-income professions. These estimates refer to the number of periodical *copies* a physician receives each month, rather than the number of different *titles*; there are four or five weekly issues of the *Journal of the American Medical Association*, for example.

As physicians become more specialized, however, the number of publications they regularly receive may be reduced. An obstetrician-gynecologist, for example, may receive only eight to 10 magazines monthly, including such periodicals as *Medical Aspects of Human Sexuality;* the *Journal of the American Medical Association; Obstetrics and Gynecology*, the official publication of the American College of Obstetricians and Gynecologists; and a few general publications.

Circulation

Magazine circulation can be either "controlled," indicating that the periodical is distributed to its recipients at no charge, or "paid," designating that the reader has paid for the magazine in order to receive it. It is easier and less expensive to launch a new magazine as a controlled publication, because controlled circulation can yield a selected group of readers, and, at the same time, eliminate the expense of securing both subscriptions and renewals.

In the magazine field, the size of the audience reached determines the rate the magazine can charge for advertising. It is difficult, costly and in most cases impossible for a paid circulation magazine to get everyone in its identifiable audience to purchase the magazine. The publisher of a controlled magazine, however, requires only the small investment necessary to assemble a mailing list of his potential audience; he can then send the publication to everyone in that audience. Thus, a controlled magazine is capable of reaching 100% of its audience.

There are also drawbacks to controlled circulation. The most significant disadvantage is that with controlled circulation the subscriber pays no part of the magazine's distribution costs. Thus, the publication's cost burden rests entirely on the advertisers, whereas a paid publication has two streams of revenue—advertising and circulation. Circulation revenue is less sensitive to economic fluctuations than advertising revenue and also provides leverage for a magazine. Some publishers feel, however, that the additional revenue obtained from paid circulation is offset by the costs of subscription acquisition.

Controlled circulation is by far the most prevalent type of circulation among medical magazines, primarily because of the ease with which lists of physicians by specialty can be secured. (Several companies are franchised by the American Medical Association to sell its lists, provided the AMA approves the mailing piece.) It should also be pointed out that, because most medical magazines are controlled, it would be extremely difficult for a new magazine to enter the field as a paid publication unless it differed significantly from existing publications.

Nursing Magazines

Nursing magazines differ from other periodicals in the medical field in that nearly all are paid circulation publications. Of the four major magazines—*Nursing '84, American Journal of Nursing, RN* and *Nursing Management*—only *Nursing Management*, with a circulation of 91,660, is controlled. Nurses have traditionally paid for their magazines, and are ostensibly willing to do so. Moreover, since most advertisers believe nurses have no influence on the selection of drugs or equipment, advertising revenues would probably be insufficient to support a controlled publication.

Advertising

The medical magazine field is one of the few business magazine fields in which syndicated audience studies are used by advertising agencies in purchasing space. Most other sectors have too diverse or too small an audience to conduct these studies economically. In addition, because the medical field is highly competitive, and most magazines are controlled, the advertiser wants proof that physicians are actually reading the magazine.

Industry observers claim physicians *do* read medical magazines, and believe that 70% to 80% of each magazine is read by every doctor who receives it. Others say the industry could probably prove a 25% exposure rating on every page of every publication.

Types of Advertising

Most medical magazines have an editorial/advertising ratio of 50%/50%. Generally, drugs and pharmaceuticals make up the largest advertising category in medical magazines, with equipment and nutritional products accounting for a much smaller volume. With the exception of publications such as *Medical Economics* and *Diversion*, which are concerned with the financial aspects of a practice and which carry automotive and travel ads, consumer advertising is relatively unimportant in the medical field, though magazines such as *Medical World News* may carry advertisements for cameras, automobiles, office equipment and other items.

Nursing magazines, on the other hand, carry little pharmaceutical or equipment advertising because nurses do not select these products. Therefore, their advertising consists mainly of personal merchandise, such as hosiery, footwear and uniforms. Recruitment advertising, a rapidly growing category, and ads for books are also carried. Magazines for nurses generally offer advertisers the choice of a hospital edition, which is received by nurses employed in hospitals and nursing homes, or a total circulation edition.

Competition with Other Advertising Media and Sales Techniques

Medical magazines' primary competitor for the advertising dollar is the detail man, a salesman employed by a pharmaceutical house to call on individual doctors. In 1980 the AMA estimated that a detail man's call on one doctor cost $110 and the cost has risen in succeeding years; the cost of a magazine's advertising message to that same doctor is much smaller. Table 4.4 illustrates the cost of delivering an advertising message to one thousand physicians via a black-and-white page in selected magazines. For the seven magazines listed, the cost-per-thousand physicians reached ranges from $24.66 in *Practical Cardiology* to $29.95 in *Medical World News*. The cost of reaching one physician by means of either of these magazines, then, would range from $.025 to $.030. A detail man's call has the advantage of direct contact with the physician on a one-to-one basis, however, and despite the fact that salary, transportation and other expenses will continue to rise, it is likely that pharmaceutical houses will remain wedded to their detail men.

Table 4.4 Cost-Per-Thousand of Selected Medical Magazines

Magazine	One Time Black-and-White Rate	Total Circulation (in thousands)	Cost-per-Thousand
Consultant	$3190	122	$26.15
Diversion	4535	176	25.77
Medical Economics	4525	168	26.93
Medical World News	3325	111	29.95
Modern Medicine	3140	120	26.17
Patient Care	3100	117	26.50
Practical Cardiology	3033	123	24.66

Source: Standard Rate & Data Service, Inc., *Business Publication Rates and Data*, July 24, 1983.

Other competitors for the medical advertising dollar include medical journals; direct mail; educational films and audio cassettes produced by pharmaceutical manufacturers; and single-sponsored publications (which will be considered later in this chapter). Video cassettes on health topics and special channels on cable television directed to doctors are also beginning to appear. In fall 1983, for example, the Cable Health Network launched Physicians' Journal Update, a two-hour satellite-delivered program for physicians that summarizes important articles in medical journals. Initially, eight major pharmaceutical companies were among the sponsors.

Economics

Starting a Magazine

The larger the interested circulation of a new medical magazine, the higher its cost. As circulation increases, costs of paper, printing, postage, etc., rise, although editorial costs remain stable regardless of circulation size.

It is difficult to start a medical magazine today because of rising costs, especially those connected with postage. A large company, such as McGraw-Hill, can sustain a postage increase, but a small entrepreneur may not be able to do so. Industry observers say the cost of launching a new magazine may range from $300,000 for a publication directed to a narrow specialty to more than $1 million for a magazine directed to general practitioners, internists and osteopaths.

Some magazines with paid circulation have been launched for much less, however. *Nursing '84*, for example, was started in 1971 with an investment of less than $50,000; revenue from initial subscriptions was plowed back into more circulation promotion.

Costs

As is true of the economy as a whole, publishing costs are constantly rising. The most dramatic increase has been in regular second-class postal costs, which have risen an average of 141% between 1973 and 1983.

The wholesale price index of paper also rose 132% between 1973 and 1983 (see Table 4.5). Paper suppliers are continuing to pass along their increased costs for items such as energy, chemicals and wages in the form of even higher prices to customers. Other items, such as printing, labor and advertising sales expenses, are also experiencing steady increases.

**Table 4.5 Wholesale Price Index of Paper, 1973-1983
(1967 = 100)**

Year	Index
1973	121.4
1974	148.6
1975	172.9
1976	182.3
1977	194.3
1978	206.1
1979	229.6
1980	256.8
1981	279.8
1982	286.3
1983	281.9
Increase, 1973-1983: 132.2%	

Source: U.S. Dept. of Labor, Bureau of Labor Statistics.

Revenue and Expense Model

It is difficult to provide meaningful averages for medical magazines because of the many differences among them with respect to circulation size, quality of paper utilized, editorial content, etc. Table 4.6, therefore, is a general model for controlled-circulation medical magazines. The revenue figures are quite different from those of consumer magazines, in which circulation revenue averages 45% of the total.

On the expense side, the model also differs in some areas from that for consumer magazines. Combined costs of circulation, distribution, paper, printing and binding are lower for medical magazines, presumably because circulations are generally smaller (leading to correspondingly smaller outlays for production and distribution) and because there are no subscription acquisition costs for controlled circulation magazines. Advertising sales expense for medical magazines, on the other hand, is nearly three times the 8% shown for consumer magazines. This is not surprising considering that advertising sales are the sole source of controlled magazine revenue.

Profitability

As is true of any advertiser-supported publication, once the break-even

Table 4.6 Revenue and Expense Model for Controlled-Circulation Medical Magazines Compared With Consumer Magazines

Financial Category	Controlled-Circulation Medical Magazines	Consumer Magazines
Revenue		
Net advertising revenue	100%	55%
Gross subscription revenue	0	30
Gross single-copy revenue	0	15
Total Revenue	100%	100%
Expense		
Circulation and distribution, paper, printing and binding	40%	65%
Advertising sales	22	8
Editorial	14	8
Other (postage, operating costs, administration)	15	10
Total Expense	91%	91%
Profit Before Taxes	9%	9%

Source: Knowledge Industry Publications, Inc.

point is reached, medical magazines can be quite profitable. The variable cost of including another five or 10 pages of advertising per issue is low; therefore, a large portion of additional advertising revenue becomes operating profit. In most cases, however, figures on the profitability of individual magazines are a closely held secret. Profit figures for individual publishers of medical magazines are of little help because they group together many types of magazines and, in some cases, combine magazine revenues with the revenues of other publishing operations. Industry experts claim that a successful trade magazine can earn 20% pretax, and some can earn as high as 30%.

Expanding the Revenue Base

As is the case with newsletters, publishers of medical magazines are also attempting to expand their revenue bases, often by recycling material that has appeared in their magazines. In addition to providing extra funds, new sources of revenue are also a means of smoothing out the erratic income flow sometimes caused by the cyclical nature of advertising. The following examples illustrate ways in which several publishers are tapping added sources of revenue.

Springhouse Corp. publishes books on nursing subjects that are marketed by direct mail as continuity series to *Nursing '84* subscribers. It also publishes an annual Career Directory, which contains some editorial material in addition to employment opportunity advertising.

Patient Care Publications publishes the *Patient Care Flow Chart Manual*, an annual hardcover publication that is sold to physicians, medical schools, etc., for $39.95. The manual contains 295 flowcharts that are logical summaries of diagnostic, therapeutic and management techniques and are a recycling of material that originally appeared in *Patient Care*. The company also produces, special flowcharts on specialized topics—e.g., the uses of a specific drug—that are marketed to pharmaceutical houses.

Medical Economics Co. publishes books on subjects covered by its magazines. It also conducts customized research and produces custom communications, such as courses, booklets and single-advertiser journals, for the pharmaceutical industry. In addition to its *Physicians' Desk Reference* and *Physicians' Desk Reference for Nonprescription Drugs*, the company also publishes several other directories in fields related to its magazines for physicians, and in April 1984 *Physicians' Desk Reference* went online as part of PHYCOM, an information service for physicians.

International Sales

Most controlled medical magazines have little or no international circulation, presumably because advertising support for foreign readership is lacking. Since the name of a drug abroad may differ from its name in the United States, advertisements in a U.S. medical magazine are often meaningless to a foreign physician, even though the periodical's editorial content may interest him or her. Thus, pharmaceutical advertisers are not interested in this type of circulation, and each country has its own network of magazines.

There are exceptions, however. For example, *Modern Medicine*, a Harcourt Brace Jovanovich publication, is produced in nine foreign editions, in the United Kingdom, Canada, West Germany, Australia, the Netherlands, South Africa, New Zealand, Ireland, and Japan. Each edition is published in the local language and carries its own advertising, although generally most of the editorial content is identical. Harcourt's *Geriatrics* magazine is published in four foreign editions, in Spain, France, Argentina and Italy. Although McGraw-Hill's domestic medical magazines have no international circulation, the company is involved in *Nikkei Medical*, a Japanese joint venture, and licenses the rights for the editorial content of *Postgraduate Medicine* to Ediciones Lerner.

Journals

Scientific research journals in printed form have been the principal mode of written communication among scientists since 1664. Journals are the vehicles of science, and as science expands into new disciplines, journals will increasingly reflect these developments.
Established journals, which have clearly defined subject boundaries, are often unable to fulfill the demands for space, attention and speed of publication that covering a new discipline would require. New groups that want to have their research published quickly, in order to receive the status and recognition that comes with publication, have found that the most rapid means of calling attention to their discipline is to establish their own journals.

The "twigging phenomenon" occurs in journal publishing in the same manner as in book publishing. In order to keep pace with the explosive growth of science over the last three decades and with the proliferation of subdisciplines, one journal may give birth to a dozen offspring. Yet the original journal continues to flourish. For example, in 1949 Plenum Publishing Corp. began translating the Russian *Journal of General Chemistry*. "Twigs" dealing with more specialized aspects of chemistry appeared rapidly; however, the original journal still exists and publishes a greater number of pages annually than it did more than 30 years ago. Thus, the number of scientific journals continues to increase as the disciplines themselves continue to expand in size and number.

Journal Circulation

Journal circulations vary tremendously and range from less than 1000 for new or very specialized publications to over 200,000 for publications such as the *New England Journal of Medicine (NEJM)* to over 300,000 for publications such as the *Journal of the American Medical Association (JAMA)*.

Because the number of small, specialized journals is far greater than the number of broad-based journals, median journal circulation is quite low. Studies by King Research, by the Indiana University School of Library Science and by researchers led by Fritz Machlup, have provided some statistics on average journal circulation. For example, a study conducted by Machlup and Leeson indicates that in 1974 the average circulation of a sample of 159 journals was 4840 copies; the median circulation of these same journals was 2430. Thus, one-half of these journals had circulations of under 2500 and, in fact, 40 of the total 159 had circulations of under 1000 copies. Small circulation does not necessarily mean lack of profitability, however, and many commercial journal publishers have journals with circulations of 5000 and under.

Subscription Acquisition

Journals are marketed to individuals and libraries, and promotional activities must be underway some time before the first issue appears. Promotion and publicity for a new journal should, in fact, begin some nine to 12 months before its initial publication. Librarians must receive information about the journal, including such specifics as its intended audience, whether and where it will be indexed, and, perhaps, a sample copy. Since most libraries order their periodicals through subscription agencies, the agencies must be made aware of forthcoming publications as soon as possible.

The cost of acquiring a subscription varies with the price of the journal, the method of acquisition, and the source through which the subscription is obtained; it is also based on whether the journal is published by a commercial or a not-for-profit publisher. Most commercial journal publishers obtain the great majority of their subscribers by direct mail. However, other methods are employed as well. Harper & Row, for example, also secures subscriptions through its salesmen who call on physicians to sell its books. Some publishers use a postage-paid order card inserted within the pages of a journal; library readers may return the card to order their own personal subscription, and the publisher only incurs a minimal cost by using this method. Publishers also exhibit at professional and library meetings or advertise in related journals.

Because society-sponsored journals have a built-in market, their subscription acquisition practices are somewhat different. Arrangements for member subscriptions to journals published by societies vary. For example, The American Chemical Society (ACS) sends its *Chemical & Engineering News* magazine to its members automatically; however, each of its 21 other publications can be purchased by members at a special subscription rate.

Members of the Institute of Electrical and Electronics Engineers (IEEE) have the option of joining one or more of its 35 member societies (which have memberships of 5000 to 10,000), thereby receiving that society's journal as part of their membership fee. If a given society publishes more than one journal, members may choose the one they wish to receive free. Nonmember subscribers to IEEE journals are generally libraries.

Members of the American Medical Association (AMA) receive *JAMA*, the weekly *American Medical News* and one of the Association's nine specialty journals in exchange for their dues. In order to receive additional journals, they must pay the periodical's regular subscription rate.

Each member of the nine societies that own and make up the American Institute of Physics (AIP) receives the Institute's *Physics Today* magazine with his or her membership. Some individual societies send their own journals automatically to every member, while others charge a special member rate. Nonmember subscriptions (mostly from libraries) are solicited by direct mail, and the majority come through subscription agencies.

The American Association for the Advancement of Science automatically sends its *Science* journal to its members in return for their dues. Individual nonmembers, as opposed to institutions, may subscribe to the magazine. Their subscription cost, however, is higher than membership dues.

The *NEJM* is automatically sent to the 11,200 members of the Massachusetts Medical Society; however, it also solicits nonmember subscriptions by direct mail and utilizes subscription agencies.

There is evidence to suggest that the practice of including a subscription to a society journal as one benefit obtained through paying membership dues may be going out of favor. An increasing number of societies appear to be initiating membership subscription rates for their journals and are giving their members the option to subscribe. If this practice becomes prevalent, it will have a major effect on subscription acquisition costs of society-sponsored publications and may lead to the demise of some journals that have small audiences.

Subscription agencies are important both to the journal publisher and to the consumer who purchases a multitude of journals, and subscriptions placed through agencies can account for a large share of a publisher's subscription volume. One publisher, for example, deals with 1700 agencies that account for about 40% of its circulation. Another, however, offers libraries consolidated billing, just as an agency does, and claims to receive fewer orders through agents than any other publisher; its average bill to a library is $20,000.

An agency usually does not solicit subscriptions for specific periodicals; instead it publishes a catalog listing the journals available and processes the orders that it receives. It charges a fee to libraries using its service, and also receives a commission from the publisher. Libraries do not want to deal with each publisher on an individual basis; paying an agency is less expensive than processing each subscription separately. Agencies are especially important in the sale of foreign subscriptions because of currency exchange problems, and one industry analyst estimates that 75% to 80% of foreign subscriptions are sold through agencies.

Many journal publishers sell subscriptions only on a calendar-year or volume-year basis; this is easier for both the library and the publisher in terms of billing, ordering and fulfillment. Some of the leading journal publishers will begin a subscription at any time, however.

Library Purchases of Journals

The proportion of journal subscriptions sold to libraries vs. individuals depends on several factors, including the price and subject of the journal and, if it is a society-sponsored publication, the number of membership subscriptions.

Williams & Wilkins, which publishes many journals priced at $35 to $60 a year, finds most of its sales are to individuals rather than to libraries. On the other hand, the AIP, which publishes several high-priced Soviet journals in translation, finds they are purchased almost entirely by libraries. In general, the more erudite the journal, the more likely it is to be purchased by libraries rather than by individuals; the larger the society that sponsors a journal, the smaller its proportion of library sales.

In the past, academic libraries relied on members of their faculties to make journal purchase decisions. Today the responsibility lies with the librarian, and the newer generation of librarians tends to perceive journals in terms of their probable use rather than their intrinsic quality. In addition, the scarcity of foreign-language skills among younger academicians has caused libraries to reduce their intake of foreign-language journals and to use the resulting savings to purchase English titles.

Academic libraries are becoming increasingly resistant to new journals, particularly those concerned with a field of knowledge that is already adequately covered, those with the greatest price increases or those in splinter fields.

Ten to 15 years ago, a new journal could in its first year be assured of 500 to 1000 subscriptions from libraries all over the world. Today, libraries do not have large budgets and are reluctant to purchase new journals. To succeed immediately, a journal must be the first in a new field, or have well-known authors as well as a prestigious editorial board and a publisher that can afford abundant promotion. Otherwise, a library may wait 18 to 36 months before making its purchase. Foreign libraries are even slower in their acceptance of new journals.

Industry observers estimate that academic libraries spend over 50%, and, in some cases, as much as 75%, of the book and periodical budgets on sci-tech journals. The costs of recording or processing each issue plus the costs of binding and shelving must be added to subscription costs. Because of the squeeze on their budgets, many libraries have shifted from book to journal acquisition simply to maintain their present journal collections. Now, however, libraries are examining subscriptions more closely and are dropping duplicate subscriptions and subscriptions to publications that are infrequently used.

Renewal Rates

Renewal rates for TSM journals are usually about 80% to 90%. (The average renewal rate for a nursing journal is probably about 60%, however, because nurses are constantly entering and leaving the work force.) The higher the renewal rate, the less the cost of subscription acquisition for the publisher of an established journal, because only a small portion of its list needs to be replaced annually.

Renewal rates are high in this field for several reasons. Individuals engaged in TSM professions find that journals are practically required reading to keep up in a field. Members may get society journals automatically, while libraries tend to renew journal subscriptions in order to maintain continuity of collections.

International Sales

The proportion of foreign to domestic subscriptions to TSM journals varies, but most journals find that 30% to 50% of their subscribers are outside the United States. This proportion will probably increase in the future as more publishers become aware of the sales potential of the international market.

The most important outlets for international sales are the English-speaking countries, Japan, Western Europe and South America. Japan, in fact, is the largest market for the export of medical information in the English language; the Japanese are affluent, aggressive and hungry for information. Although not an important market at present, China is expected by many journal publishers to become a significant market in the future.

Most journals are printed in English regardless of their destination. Some publishers will occasionally print the abstract of an article in a foreign language; however, this practice is being phased out, both because of its expense and because English has become the language of the scientist. The AMA, however, believing that the average foreign physician finds his own language more comfortable than English, publishes *JAMA* in French, Japanese, German, Flemish, Italian and Chinese.

Journal Translations

Because most American scientists do not read Russian or Chinese, they find it necessary to have journals in these languages translated into English. The AIP and Plenum Publishing Corp. are probably the two journal publishers doing the most work in this area.

The AIP publishes 60% of Soviet physics research in 19 publications that are translations of Soviet journals; their worldwide circulations range from 400 to 1200. In addition, in 1981 the AIP began publishing *Chinese Physics*, a quarterly which contains translations of the best articles from 13 Chinese physics and astronomy journals.

Plenum's Consultants Bureau division, established in 1949, publishes the largest number of English translations of Soviet scientific books and journals in the world. English translations of 95 Soviet journals are published under its Consultants Bureau imprint; it also has a contract with a learned society whereby it produces translations of 11 Soviet journals for publication by that society.

ECONOMICS OF JOURNAL PUBLISHING

Although the economics of commercial and society-sponsored journal publishing are similar in most respects, there are some aspects of publishing that apply only to the latter. This section covers the economics of journal publishing that are common to both groups; the following section discusses those elements unique to society-sponsored journals.

Starting a New Journal

In order to enjoy a fairly good chance of success, a new journal should ideally be started in a dynamic, emerging new area in which there is little or no competition. The institutions conducting research in the field must be identified, and the publisher should know the number of people actively working in or interested in the field. An editor in chief with contacts and prestige, and a committed editorial board that will help in the search for high-grade papers are also necessary. Perhaps most important, there must be a sufficient flow of good papers. Ordinarily, a new journal must compete with existing journals for such papers. (One publisher says that a journal that cannot maintain a regular publication pattern of at least four issues a year is doomed to failure.) A rapid schedule for publication is necessary; it should take no more than six months from a paper's receipt until its final publication. A publisher must also consider the journal's advertising potential, competition from other journals and potential reprint income from authors and corporations that will want to use an article which they feel mentions their product in a favorable manner.

The potential worldwide market for a journal approximates the number of people working in the field, although in today's world of library networking and photocopying, it is unlikely that a publisher will ever reach the full potential market. One journal publisher has stated that the potential market for a journal should be equal to four times the number of subscribers at its break-even point, or the publication will not succeed. The problem with this formula lies in determining the size of the potential market.

It is difficult to start a new journal today because, in most cases, there is so much competition. There are exceptions, however, in the case of some highly specialized areas. For example, in 1976 Mosby began *The Journal of Hand Surgery*, the official journal of the American Society for Surgery of the Hand. Mosby had been asked by the society since the early 1970s to publish such a title; at that time the society had 150 to 200 members, and the publisher felt the timing was wrong. After certain microsurgical advances occurred which needed to be communicated, Mosby decided to go ahead with publication. The journal now has 7400 subscribers worldwide. Many industry experts feel, however, that there are few such opportunities left.

It may cost anywhere from $10,000 to more than $50,000 to launch a journal. The actual costs depend on many factors, including the subject area, existing competition, the number of other journals produced by the publisher, the number of library subscribers to the publisher's other journals, whether it is a society-sponsored publication and the printing processes employed.

If a company publishes several journals, there are economies with respect to overhead, personnel, paper and printing costs, etc., that can make a new journal less costly. Moreover, if the publisher has a large number of existing library subscribers, it can easily promote a new journal to them. In addition, a society-sponsored journal has a built-in market among members. Finally, a journal can be launched at a relatively low cost by having authors submit camera-ready copy, or it can use glossy paper, illustrations, and other costly items and be extremely expensive.

The success of a journal is linked to growth of the field it covers, and the publication will live as long as the field survives. A journal in a rapidly changing segment of science may have a short life span. On the other hand, a journal in a field that is large and growing may split into several journals.

Publishers today cannot start a journal in a basic science and hope the field will grow; these fields are already developed. As a result, many journals are begun in minor scientific areas in the hope that they will grow into major scientific fields.

The Break-even Point

Most publishers expect that it will take from three to five years for a journal to break even. Some publishers have waited as long as nine years to reach the break-even point, however; others do not launch a journal unless they expect it to show a profit at the close of its first year.

The break-even point for a specific journal depends on its cost (especially as regards the type of production involved—camera-ready or other) and its price. The higher the production cost, the longer it will take to break even. As for the price, the higher the price (within limits), the shorter the time period required to break even.

Reaching break-even should be easier for the multijournal publisher who does not need to add overhead when he adds a new journal. Realistically, only the out-of-pocket expenses that can be directly attributed to the new journal are relevant; they way in which fixed costs are allocated to a new journal should be strictly an accounting matter. Thus, if a publication is breaking even before it is allocated a share of general and administrative overhead, it is paying its way.

Costs

Journals can be expensive to produce. Not every subject lends itself to the use of camera-ready copy and inexpensive paper. Some fields utilize many formulas and tables; in such cases, glossy paper is required in order to reproduce illustrations successfully. Illustrations, tables or formulas can more than triple or quadruple charges; composition costs for a page of straight text can be $6, as opposed to $40 for a page of complex formulas, for example. Thus, journal publishing costs may vary according to the subject.

Postage has also become a costly item. Nearly all publishers charge for postage and handling outside the United States. Some publishers also charge for domestic copies, but usually their charge is less than the actual cost.

It is difficult to find ways in which costs can be reduced, especially since publishers try to do so in areas that will not affect a journal's quality. Although a journal publisher can change to camera-ready copy or eliminate outside editing, doing so may affect the quality of the publication. Similarly, computerized typesetting does not greatly reduce expenses because it does not affect many of the major costs, such as paper, binding, distribution and agency discounts.

Pricing and Price Elasticity

For the most part, the journal market is not sensitive to price; therefore, when a journal raises its price, it may not lose more than a few subscribers. What price sensitivity there is depends to a great extent upon journal quality, competition, the subject matter and the proportion of library subscribers. The market for a high-quality journal is virtually inelastic; the journal is practically required reading, since advances in a specific field will be chronicled in a journal much sooner than in a book, which may take 12 to 18 months before publication. If there is another journal in the same field, however, a subscriber may choose the less expensive of the two, if he or she feels they are equal in quality. Journals in the social sciences or in the humanities tend to be much more price-sensitive than those in the hard sciences, such as physics and chemistry.

A journal with a large proportion of library subscribers will tend to be much less sensitive to price than a journal with many individual subscribers. A library subscriber has made a conscious decision to subscribe to a particular journal, and a price increase will not change this decision. Libraries also try to maintain the continuity of their collections and are reluctant to cancel journal subscriptions. Moreover, many of them build an inflation factor into their budgets to cover price increases. Thus, a society-sponsored journal with a large proportion of libraries as nonmember subscribers will have an extremely inelastic market. Its members probably receive the publication as part of their dues or at a special rate, and its library subscribers will generally tend to renew, regardless of price.

Limitations to journal prices are imposed both by competition and by the nature of the market. It would be dangerous, for example, to price a journal significantly higher than the prevailing charge in the social sciences, biology or geology because journals in these fields have traditionally enjoyed government support. The market is not as price-sensitive in biochemistry, biophysics and other interdisciplinary fields, while subscription prices can be tied to true costs in the physical and life sciences, medicine, engineering and some earth sciences.

Influence of Federal Funding

A large proportion of research in TSM fields is subsidized by the federal government. Although government funding has an effect on the type of research that is conducted and, therefore, published, it is not the only influence; funding may also be obtained from private sources. In any case, a journal publisher should be aware of those fields the government is funding as well as those fields in which research funds are drying up.

Federal funding has an even more direct effect on journal publishing than simply determining the types of research being conducted. Research is worthless if it is not reported. Because the government recognizes this, its grants provide for publication expenses, such as reprints and page charges. Sometimes government funding also aids subscription sales; the recipient of a government grant, for example, may use it to order a new journal subscription, which his library may continue after the grant runs out.

Advertising

Sci-tech journals usually carry little advertising, probably because their circulations are so small; most publishers claim that less than 1% of their journal revenues are derived from advertising. Those sci-tech journals that receive a relatively large amount of advertising are usually the broad-based, more general publications, such as *Science*. Most advertisements are for instrumentation or for books and journals issued by other publishers, and advertisements for the latter are often carried on an exchange basis.

In contrast to sci-tech journals, many medical journals carry a great deal of advertising; most leading medical journal publishers say advertising accounts for 20% to 35% of their total revenue. The amount of advertising revenue depends on the subject matter of the publication, its resulting audience and the size of its circulation. The AMA's *Archives of Pathology and Laboratory Medicine,* for example, carries no drug advertising because pathologists do not prescribe drugs. Its *Archives of Internal Medicine,* on the other hand, deals in several areas of medicine and carries a great deal of advertising. In general, the more "vertical" or specialized a journal, the better its potential for advertising revenue because the advertiser can be more certain of reaching his desired prospects. This axiom does not always hold true, however; the *NEJM,* which, according to *Folio,* carried about $9.9 million of advertising revenue in 1982, attributes its success to its broad appeal. Presumably, this would be true also of *JAMA,* which carried $12.3 million of advertising in 1982, according to *Folio.*

Medical journals face competition for advertising from controlled circulation magazines, which, since they are sent free to everyone in a field, can offer more comprehensive coverage for the advertiser. The most important categories for medical advertising are surgical and X-ray equipment, other medical instruments and devices, books, employment advertising, retirement plans, ethical drugs and some proprietary drugs. Medical journals carry little advertising for consumer products.

Journals that carry little advertising may have a ratio of 97% editorial material to 3% advertising. Those carrying heavy advertising may have a 55% to 45% ratio, but the average is probably 65% to 70% editorial material to 30% to 35% advertising.

The *NEJM* appears to be the only major medical journal that publishes a regional edition. Its New England regional edition is published once a month. Editorial content is identical to that of the regular edition, but each issue contains local advertising from hospital suppliers, banks, real estate brokers, etc.

Profitability

A successful journal can be profitable for several reasons. Once a journal has been established, and there is a prescribed system for submitting articles, little investment is required. Manuscripts are submitted by outside writers, and only a small staff of editors, some of them free-lancers, is required to prepare articles for publication. Once an audience is acquired, a journal must still continue to promote itself, but a large core of subscribers will renew year after year. Therefore, promotion expense can be minimal.

A journal receives its subscription income a year in advance. Although it is treated in accounting terms as "unearned income,"[4] it is also cash on hand; the publisher earns interest on it, and the journal is produced with someone else's money.

Advertising provides leverage for a journal. Most journals are designed to make money from circulation, so advertising results in extra revenues at relatively little additional cost.

Economies of scale also are involved in multijournal publishing and greatly enhance profitability. These economies result from better use of staff: one person usually can be responsible for the editorial, advertising or fulfillment activities of several journals. Production and fulfillment costs per publication are usually reduced in multijournal publishing, and overhead costs can be spread over several units.

---

[4] A publisher who receives a $100 check in December for a subscription starting January 1 will show a liability on its balance sheet of $100 in "unearned income" as of December 31. In each succeeding quarter, the publisher will recognize $25 as subscription revenue, thus reducing its liability by that amount.

Revenue and Expense Model

It is difficult to provide meaningful averages for TSM journals because of the many differences among them. The basic differences lie in advertising volume and the type of publisher (i.e., a not-for-profit organization or a commercial publisher). However, differences in circulation size, quality and quantity of paper used, use of formulas and illustrations, and publication frequency are also among the factors that make it difficult to present meaningful figures.

Table 4.7 is a general model for a commercial journal in the medical field, and the revenue figures therefore differ from those of a sci-tech journal, which presumably would have advertising revenues of about 1%. The proportions of subscription sales revenues and order fulfillment costs are also higher than they would be if the model were for a society-sponsored journal for which the subscription is automatically included in the dues.

Journal Publishing by Book Publishing Houses

Many journal publishers, such as Mosby, Raven Press and John Wiley & Sons, are also book publishers. The advantages of journal publishing should be carefully examined by a book publishing house as another form of publishing with which the company might become involved. Journal publishing can be quite profitable, and because subscription payments are received in advance these funds can be used to finance books at interest-free rates. In addition, journal publishing gives a book publisher contact with potential book authors who are currently journal contributors.

ECONOMICS OF JOURNAL PUBLISHING FOR SOCIETY-SPONSORED JOURNALS

Not-for-Profit vs. Commercial Publishers

Not-for-profit journals and commercial journals differ in that each has a different audience mix, a different financial base and a different motive for publishing.

Commercial journals tend to be distributed primarily to libraries, with relatively few individual subscriptions; the preponderance of circulation for society-sponsored journals is to individuals, with library subscribers in the minority. The library populations are probably similar in both types of publishing, but societies are less dependent on libraries for subscription income.

Table 4.7 Revenue and Expense Model for a Commercially Published Journal in the Basic Sciences[1]

Financial Category	Component as Percent of Total
Revenue	
Subscription sales	73%
Advertising sales	17
Other (back copies, reprints, rights, mailing lists, microfilm, etc.)	10
Total Revenue	100%
Expense	
Cost of Sales	
Manufacturing costs	
Text	37%
Advertising	5
Other (reprints, microfilm)	4
Editorial and redactory costs	7
Overhead (journal management and advertising production)	3
Total Cost of Sales	56%
Selling and Distribution Costs	
Shipping and storage	7%
Subscription sales overhead	2
Order fulfillment	5
Sales commissions (advertising, microfilm, mailing list)	3
Total Selling and Distribution Costs	17%
Administrative and General Overhead	5%
Total Expenses	78%
Profit Before Taxes	22%

[1] Assumes that the journal is the official publication of a prestigious society in the basic medical sciences; member subscriptions comprise less than 20% of the total. Average subscription rate is approximately $29. Publication is a monthly with a circulation of 4485 and 885 pages of text per year.
Source: Knowledge Industry Publications, Inc., based on industry sources.

A not-for-profit publisher is exempt from some taxes (such as income tax) and can mail at a lower postage rate than a commercial publisher. Such a publisher may charge for publication of submitted material;

sometimes it may also produce a magazine (such as IEEE does with *Spectrum*) that charges higher rates for advertising and consequently helps to subsidize its journal publishing operation. Because the journal is usually sent to society members automatically, a not-for-profit publisher has a guaranteed circulation and low subscription-acquisition costs. In addition, it does not have stockholders, and therefore does not need to produce a net profit. As a result, it can price its journals at a level that allows them to break even and perhaps cover some of the costs of society operations.

The basic publishing motive of a not-for-profit publisher is to serve the needs of its members rather than to make a profit (which is the goal of the commercial publisher). Thus, a not-for-profit publisher need not consider the wishes of advertisers, e.g., in its arrangement of advertising and editorial copy. A not-for-profit publisher may also be more willing to do a journal in an important, but marginally profitable, field. It should also be noted that the publisher of a society-sponsored journal has access to and can print all the papers presented at society meetings—presumably the best of the research currently being conducted. Competitive commercial publishers normally do not have access to these papers.

Society-Sponsored Journals Published by Commercial Publishers

When a society-sponsored journal is published by a commercial publisher, the editor, who is usually a society employee or member, is responsible for its editorial content. The publisher receives material from the editor and takes over all other responsibilities for producing the journal. Financial arrangements vary, but generally the publisher collects all reprint, subscription and advertising income and pays all bills, including editorial charges. The publisher recovers his direct cost, adds on something for overhead and divides the net profit, if there is any, with the society; if there is a loss, the publisher suffers it alone. In addition, the publisher often pays the society a sum of money as a stipend for permitting his company to produce the journal whether or not it shows a profit. Thus, the society has a no-risk arrangement. In some recent instances, societies have become more interested in a guaranteed income than in a share of the profits. As a result, they have negotiated for fixed dollars, a percent of revenues, or a guaranteed minimum against a percent of revenue.

When a society is small or has only one journal, it is usually more profitable for the society-sponsored journal to be published by a commercial publisher than by the society itself. A society would need staff to carry out all the functions provided by the commercial publisher. The commercial publisher usually manages the journal more efficiently than the society, and achieves economies of scale if it publishes other journals.

Page Charges

In the late 1920s, the American Physical Society incurred financial problems in publishing *The Physical Review*. A committee formed to study the problem noted that "institutions supporting research can justly be asked to bear a portion of the cost of the publication of results," suggesting a charge of $2 per published page. In this manner, the policy of page charges was begun.

There are many arguments that can be advanced in order to justify a page charge policy:

• No research can be considered complete until its results are a matter of record. Since processing a manuscript for publication is costly, it is fair to ask those who support research to assist financially in its publication; most research is done on grants, and funds for publication are generally included.

• Journal publication serves not only the reader but also the author and his or her institution by aiding in their advancement and recognition. Therefore, it is fair to ask them to contribute to the cost of this service.

• Page charges subsidize the input of publishing and make it possible to publish journals at lower subscription rates and larger circulations than journals lacking this support.

• Societies in the basic sciences try to keep their dues at minimum levels in order to attract members. Yet a page of their journals costs the same to produce as any other journal. To offset these charges which their dues structures cannot support, the societies use page charges.

The AIP, probably the most important proponent of page charges, divides publishing costs into those for editorial work and composition, and those for printing and distribution. The cost of editorial work and composition varies with the number of pages involved, but is independent of the number of copies printed. The cost of printing and distribution (which includes subscription fulfillment) is proportional to the number of subscriptions, as well as the number of pages. The AIP tailors publication income to publication costs by adjusting page charges to cover the costs of editorial work and composition and setting subscription rates to cover printing and distribution costs.

Page-charge plans appear most often in the physics field and, to some extent, in chemistry, engineering and medicine. They are most prevalent in society-sponsored journals, since the federal government will only permit charges to be paid to a not-for-profit publisher. Page charges range from as low as $20 per page to as high as $120 per page. These charges are usually voluntary rather than mandatory. Publishing decisions are generally made without knowing whether a request for payment of page charges will be honored. After an article's acceptance, the sponsoring institution is approached to pay page charges, but the article will be published whether or not the charges are paid. The AIP, however, will delay a paper's scheduled publication date by three months if page charges are not honored.

In 1977, the U.S. Postal Service ruled that editorial material supported by authors' fees (page charges) was advertising and should be so labeled by journals wishing to enjoy second-class postage rates. Pressure was exerted by the industry, however, and the ruling was reversed.

Other Charges

Some journal publishers levy one or several other types of charges on their contributors, including a nominal submission fee, a charge for manuscripts that exceed certain page limits, or charges for any illustrations, "excessive" illustrations or color illustrations.

Tax-Exempt Status

In 1970, the Internal Revenue Service (IRS) ruled that all tax-exempt or nonprofit organizations must pay a tax on net profit from advertising carried in their journals because advertising is an unrelated business. This ruling, of course, has little effect on journals in the sci-tech area because they carry so little advertising; however, for some medical journals the sums are sizable.

EXPANDING THE REVENUE BASE

There are many methods by which a journal publisher can expand its revenue, including back number sales, reprints, collections and database publishing. Back number sales are rarely significant, however, and depend on the age of a journal, its archival nature, the proportion of library subscriptions it has and the number of new library subscriptions it acquires each year.

Sales of reprints to authors are a good source of revenue; however, demand varies and is often related to the availability of grant money. Sometimes commercial sales of reprints, stimulated by the favorable mention of a company's drugs or instrumentation, prove to be quite lucrative.

Some publishers recycle their material by publishing collections of previously printed articles. The *NEJM* has several collections of its Drug Therapy columns in print. Despite the fact that they were composed of "old" material, the first four collections sold 10,000 sets at $14 each in the first three years after publication. Other publishers have had only limited success with this method, however.

The AIP places citations and abstracts of all its published articles on SPIN, an online database; and the AMA is involved in database publishing through its Medical Information Network and MED/MAIL, an electronic mail system.

Continuing Medical Education (CME)

Many journals in the medical and nursing fields are publishing materials to assist their readers in meeting continuing medical education (CME) requirements. Usually, the CME feature consists of an article accompanied by a test; some publishers process the test and keep records for the participants, while others contract with an outside agency for this service. Mosby's *Journal of the American Academy of Dermatology*, for example, publishes a CME program, and the company has had requests for more such programs. The journal's lead article is a review based on the Academy's Core Curriculum of Clinical Dermatology and is accompanied by a questionnaire which is returned to the academy by the physician.

In a variation on the usual CME programs, the American College of Physicians publishes the Medical Knowledge Self-Assessment Program, a home-study course. The program, which is reissued every three years, consists of a syllabus containing a compact review of the essential medical literature published during the preceding three years. During the first year the physician answers questions based on the materials and is sent the results (as compared to those of his or her peers) in addition to an answer book; in succeeding years, the physician must score himself. The program costs $225 for nonmembers, $125 for members and Fellows, and $85 for associates.

PROBLEMS IN JOURNAL PUBLISHING

The major problems faced by the journal industry today are the shrinking library market, the increasing competition provided by abstracting and database services, and photocopying of journal articles.

Probably the biggest problem in the journal industry is the inelastic market faced by journal publishers whose income depends primarily on library subscriptions. While the number of journals is increasing, reflecting the growth of information and research, the total amount libraries must expend to keep up with new and existing journals has gone beyond their ability to pay, and money has been diverted from book budgets. This is a situation that cannot continue much longer. Libraries will either cut back on multiple subscriptions or cancel lesser-used journals, resulting in the demise of some existing journals. Those that remain in business will be forced to raise their prices to make up for reduced circulation, and this, in turn, will lead to further cancellations.

Journals have an obligation to disseminate information; while abstracting and database services assist in this respect, on balance they are not an asset to the journal industry. Both the journals and the services are vying for the same library dollar. Now that the services are online, users tend to conduct more online searches rather than purchase the journal itself, finding that through networks they can more easily locate the material without subscribing to the journal. This, of course, reduces the circulation of the journal.

Photocopying

Photocopying of journal articles is a problem of long standing in the journal industry, and until the passage of the Copyright Act of 1976 (most sections of which became effective on January 1, 1978) there were no laws expressly addressing this problem.

In a case brought before the U.S. Court of Claims in the early 1970s—*Williams & Wilkins Co. v. U.S.*—the publisher sought copyright infringement damages with respect to the article photocopying practices of the National Library of Medicine (NLM) and the National Institute of Health (NIH). The initial judge ruled that copyright infringement did exist; however, the full Court of Claims voted 4-3 in favor of no infringement. The case went to the U.S. Supreme Court where the full court ruling was upheld by a 4-4 decision with no opinions issued.

Some of the conclusions underlying the decision of the Court of Claims were that: 1) Williams & Wilkins did not show it was being "harmed substantially"; 2) NIH and NLM are nonprofit institutions and therefore realized no gains as a result of the photocopying; 3) both libraries enforced "reasonably strict" limitations that kept the duplication "within appropriate confines"; and 4) in the period before legislative guidance is forthcoming for this type of problem, severe restrictions should not be placed on the distribution of medical research.

In 1980, Theodore Caris, publisher of Aspen Systems Corp., requested that the Copyright Office investigate the current photocopying practices of government libraries, especially NIH and NLM, as part of its five-year review of the Copyright Act of 1976. Caris believed NIH and NLM were systematically supplying photocopies of copyrighted material to interested parties without securing permission and without paying royalties, just as Williams & Wilkins claimed when they instituted their suit. Neither of these institutions is registered with the Copyright Clearance Center, nor were publishers of medical journals receiving photocopying permission requests from these institutions.

Many technological developments affecting copyrights emerged or became significant during the period between the issuance of the copyright laws of 1909 and 1976; e.g., radio, motion pictures, television, computers and photocopiers all became realities within these 67 years. The Copyright Law of 1976 attempted to deal with these developments and contained more detailed and explicit provisions concerning the right to use copyrighted works without permission. Among the new provisions were those relating to reproduction rights of libraries.

Section 108 of the Copyright Law of 1976 permits eligible libraries to reproduce and distribute a copy of a copyrighted work without the permission of the copyright owner and without infringement of copyright under certain circumstances. In order to exercise its rights under Section 108, a library's collections must be open to the public. If this is not the case, a library is still eligible to exercise these rights if its collections are available not only to researchers connected with the library, or the institution of which it is a part, but also to others performing research in a specialized field. The rights under Section 108 apply only to copies made or distributed "without any purpose of direct or indirect commercial advantage." Authorization is given only to reproduce a single copy of a specific work on one occasion, although a subsequent copy may be made on one or more "separate" occasions.

Thus, an eligible library may under certain circumstances make and distribute a copy of an article at a user's request, but this right does not extend to cases in which the library engages in "the systematic reproduction or distribution of single or multiple copies." This provision was designed to prevent the substitution of reproduced material for purchased subscriptions. CONTU (the National Commission on New Technological Uses of Copyrighted Works) developed guidelines for interlibrary arrangements, but these guidelines only pertain to articles appearing in issues published within five years prior to the date of an interlibrary request. If during a given calendar year the requesting library receives a total of no more than five copies of articles (the same article or a combination of different articles) from recent issues of the same publication, the library is within the guidelines; the sixth copy, however, goes beyond the guidelines.

In 1977 the Association of American Publishers and the Information

Industry Association formed the Copyright Clearance Center (CCC) in an attempt to deal with the problem of photocopying. Publishers participating in the CCC authorize users to copy articles in return for a fee designated by the publisher. Participating users make their copies themselves, pay the fees to the Center, and provide the Center with information on what was copied. The Center distributes the fees to the publisher based on the data supplied by the user. In 1983 the CCC initiated a new system, the Annual Authorizations Service, under which the user makes a single annual payment to CCC for a license and authorization to make all the copies needed for internal use during the year. The user does not need to record or report copying activity to CCC except during an audit period.

Despite improvements in the reporting of photocopying violations to the CCC, the number of copies reported each month was estimated in mid-1983 to be only 5% of the actual monthly volume of serial photocopying in the United States. If correct, this figure indicates widespread noncompliance, and if the CCC is to be considered successful, the number of infringements reported must increase significantly. As of late 1983 the CCC had 750 participating publishers, over 750 registered journal and book titles and 1800 registered users; the number of photocopies reported each month had reached the 30,000 to 40,000 level.

In January 1983 the Office of Copyright submitted to Congress the first five-year review of the effectiveness of photocopying provisions in the Copyright Law of 1976, focusing particularly on photocopying in libraries. The report called for the law to be amended to grant publishers more protection for their copyrighted works and asked that stricter guidelines be imposed for copying in libraries. Results of the King Research Inc. report on photocopying practices in libraries and archives, which was contracted for by the Copyright Office, indicated that 25% of all library photocopying transactions involved two or more copies and 10% involved five copies or more. In reaction to the report, the AAP proposed an "umbrella statute," which would allow users to pay a single reasonable fee for copying protected works; the statute would apply only to scientific, medical, technical and business journals and conference proceedings. The report also indicated that publishers lost $38.6 million in revenue in 1980 because of multiple photocopying; as much as $27 million of this may have been lost by publishers of sci-tech journals. These publishers received only $665,000 in photocopy royalty revenues from all sources.

OUTLOOK FOR TSM MAGAZINES AND JOURNALS

Magazines

The outlook for medical magazines must be viewed in the context of broader trends in the health communications and publishing field. Magazines are not the primary means of disseminating research findings or clinical information (journals and monographs both play this role), but they can give a broader perspective on the world of medicine, as well as provide practical information on finances and management of a practice. Basically, however, the proliferation of these magazines reflects the need of drug companies to reach the physician with drug advertising. The print medium is a relatively low-cost means of reaching physicians with advertising, even though costs have skyrocketed in the past decade.

If the threat to journals comes from computer-based information retrieval, making possible on-demand display of clinical and research data, the threat to magazines comes from yet another form of electronic publishing: audiovisual programs. Audio cassettes, films, and now video cassettes, discs and cable TV programs are all appealing methods of conveying health information. Television, in particular, is widely used and accepted by doctors as a way of showing clinical situations, real patients, or actual operations. Sponsored video programs offer advertisers a way to reach physicians without the clutter of magazine advertising. It is true that the expense of video production is high, but distribution costs are coming down as the price of video tape declines, and as the video disc becomes more widely available. Hence, it is unlikely that medical magazines will retain their present share of drug companies' advertising and promotion budgets, although the magazines should continue to grow in absolute terms.

Journals

Because journals are the primary vehicles for the communication of new information, journal publishing will continue to grow as the knowledge base expands. Placing the full text of a journal article—or an entire journal—online may become the future method for the rapid dissemination of data, especially during the period before the journal is printed and distributed. The journal will not die out, however, because researchers will still find the convenient format and portability of a journal preferable to sitting in front of a terminal and reading a printout or words on a screen. A journal can also be kept for constant reference as opposed to a database that must be accessed whenever needed.

Photocopying will still continue to be a problem for journal publishers, but perhaps additional laws will be enacted that will help to alleviate the problem.

Publishing costs will continue to increase during the next few years, resulting in rising subscription prices, which in turn will lead to a smaller library market. As a result, some journals may become economically unfeasible to produce, and new journals will find it increasingly difficult to establish themselves; however, there will always be a market for the quality and prestige publications.

OTHER PERIODICALS

Two other forms of periodicals are common in the medical segment of the TSM industry: single-advertiser magazines and "clinic"-type publications.

Single-Advertiser Magazines

Single-advertiser magazines are controlled-circulation publications that usually contain eight to 12 pages of editorial material tailored to an advertiser's market, plus a four-page advertising insert bought and paid for by one company. The editorial content of a specific issue is identical for every reader who receives a copy, but the advertising will differ depending on the reader's specialty. There is only one advertiser to an issue, however, and each magazine is distributed only to the market defined by that advertiser.

Several publishers are currently involved in this field, including the Medical Economics Co. and the CPC Communications division of Cliggot Publishing Co., publisher of *Consultant*. However, Sieber & McIntyre, a health-care communications and marketing company, pioneered this concept in 1968 in order to provide its clients with a means of communicating to a targeted audience especially interested in their messages. It is now the largest U.S. publisher of single-advertiser magazines, publishing some 50 of these periodicals in the health-care field, including *Physician's Financial Letter, Current Concepts in Trauma Care* and *Economic Disclosure*.

The circulation of Sieber & McIntyre's single-advertiser publications, most of which are quarterlies, ranges between 20,000 and 50,000 copies. An exception is *Physician's Financial Letter*, the only biweekly, which has a circulation of nearly 120,000. The editorial/advertising ratio of the company's publications is 70% editorial to 30% advertising. Costs to the advertiser range from 14 cents a copy to $1.60 a copy; they vary with the circulation and include editorial material, advertising, mailing labels, handling and postage. Sieber & McIntyre has established similar publications in the Far East, United Kingdom, Scandinavia and Europe. The editorial material for most of these magazines is produced in the country of publication, and the advertiser is located in that country as well.

Clinics and Similar Publications

W.B. Saunders Co. is the publisher of 24 Clinics of North America—hardcover periodicals published three to six times a year, containing eight to 12 articles on a specific topic. The Clinics, with titles such as *Dental Clinics of North America* or *Otolaryngologic Clinics of North America,* are sold on a subscription basis and carry no advertising; subscription prices range from $22 to $64 and single issues can be purchased at premium rates.

Clinics are considered neither magazine nor journals and perhaps most closely resemble a continuity series, except that a subscriber purchases them on an annual basis rather than paying for each title individually.

Saunders chooses a special topic for each issue of a Clinic and keeps the issues of uniform size. Each issue has a separate consulting editor who selects contributors. There is no peer review; the editor is chosen on the basis of his expertise in the subject matter, and the authors are invited to contribute papers. The authors are not paid, but each receives a free copy of the issue and about 250 reprints of his contribution. The articles are generally review articles rather than reports of original laboratory research.

In a similar type of program, Year Book publishes seven periodicals, including *Disease-A-Month* and *Current Problems in Pediatrics.* The purpose of these publications is to provide physicians with a short, concise article on a topic related to their practice. Each issue is devoted exclusively to a single topic of major importance, which in some cases may be continued from one month to the next. The articles do not consist of original research; rather, they are summaries of research and its applications to a practice. Each issue usually contains only one article (about 60 to 80 pages in length). The articles are solicited and there is no peer review as such. However, an editorial board chooses the topics and reviews the articles.

Harper & Row also publishes four clinic-type publications which are similar to those published by Saunders.

5

Newsletters and Loose-Leaf Services

Newsletters and loose-leaf services are the smallest segment of the technical, scientific and medical (TSM) information market. In 1982 they totaled $54 million, with newsletters accounting for $48 million and loose-leaf services for the remainder.

A newsletter is a concise periodical directed to a special-interest group; it is sold by subscription only and ordinarily contains no advertising. Because it summarizes and condenses, leaving details, in-depth coverage and illustrations to other media such as books, magazines or journals, an eight-page newsletter is often able to furnish as much hard information as a 70-page magazine aimed at the identical audience. The psychological advantage of a newsletter is that the user need read only a few pages on a regular basis to keep up with new developments in his or her field. (In the TSM field, however, a newsletter subscriber wishing to act on developments in his or her profession would ordinarily require more information than that presented in the newsletter alone.) Finally, newsletters provide information readers cannot obtain so quickly elsewhere, but which they need for decision and action.

A newsletter can be classified by the type of information it provides or by its price and circulation. Generally, a newsletter contains either tactical or strategic information. Tactical information is the data that the recipient absolutely requires to perform his or her job. An example of a tactical newsletter is *The Medical Letter*, which evaluates new drugs for physicians and claims to be the medical practitioner's only source of drug information that is not related to the drug industry. Strategic newsletters include those that are analytical plus those that cover news and, sometimes, gossip about the field with which they are concerned. *Science and Government Report*, which contains both scientific news of interest to government and government news of interest to scientists, falls into this category. Also included in this group are letters such as Predicasts' *Technology Update*, which presents abstracts of articles reporting on new developments in all the major technological fields.

Most newsletters tend to be sold either at a high price with low circulation (specialized areas) or at a low price with high circulation (more general areas). The TSM field includes both categories of letters.

A loose-leaf reference service is simply what its name suggests—a reference volume or volumes on a specific topic presented in some type of binder so that it may be updated on a regular basis as new developments occur. Few of these services are published for the TSM field, and their estimated total revenue in 1982 was about $6 million.

COMPARISON OF NEWSLETTERS WITH MAGAZINES AND JOURNALS

Several differences exist between newsletters and magazines; however, there are both similarities and differences between newsletters and journals.

Newsletters and Magazines

The most obvious difference between newsletters and magazines in the TSM field (and that upon which most other differences depend) is that generally newsletters do not accept advertising. Thus, newsletters are supported by subscription revenue plus the sale of any related services or products. This is in contrast to magazines, many of which—especially in the medical area—are sent to their subscribers at no charge and depend on advertising revenue as their sole source of income. Revenue from advertising is usually the major source of income even for those publications that charge a subscription fee. Thus, for newsletters the total cost of publication is passed on to the subscriber, whereas magazines charge their readers only a fraction of their publishing costs.

Reflecting this situation, newsletter prices are generally higher than magazine prices. The higher prices can be justified by the highly specialized subject matter they contain. (This often creates a problem for a newsletter just entering the market, however, because prospective readers do not always understand the reasons for its high subscription rate.)

Launching a newsletter does not require as large an investment as starting a magazine. All its revenue is up front in the form of subscription fees, while magazines do not receive their advertising revenue until after the advertising has appeared. In addition, a newsletter must only please its subscribers, in contrast to a magazine, which must satisfy its advertisers as well as its readers. Finally, publishers may have less flexibility in raising advertising rates than in boosting the price of a specialized newsletter.

Newsletters and Journals

There are both similarities and differences between newsletters and journals. The major difference between the two is in editorial content. A newsletter usually carries up-to-the-minute, concise information on current developments in a field. A journal, on the other hand, contains in-depth scholarly papers on research findings in a specific area, which have been reviewed before publication by experts in the field.

Although newsletters generally do not accept advertising, journals are often supported by a combination of subscription and advertising revenue. The proportion of advertising varies with the subject matter of the journal. Medical journals, for example, carry a great deal, but many journals serving the scientific and technical (sci-tech) areas carry little or none.

Newsletters are generally produced by an individual entrepreneur or commercial publisher and must show a profit to survive. Many journals, on the other hand, are sponsored by nonprofit organizations and are not expected to make a profit. In the frequent instances in which a society-sponsored journal is published by a commercial publisher, the publisher usually shoulders any losses that may occur, while the society gets a royalty or share of any profits; thus, in this case, the society has a no-risk publication.

Journals are similar to newsletters in that they often also require only a small investment to begin publication. A sizable portion, if not all, of their revenue is up front in the form of subscription fees. In addition, journals generally do not pay for their editorial material—in fact, they may charge the author a fee for its publication—and may be started with an editorial staff of only one person.

Like newsletters, journals are often able to charge high prices for subscriptions. Many subscriptions are purchased by libraries that try to continue their purchases, despite rate increases, in order to maintain a complete series. (Budget cuts have nevertheless forced libraries to prune journal subscriptions.)

SIZE AND STRUCTURE OF THE NEWSLETTER MARKET

Because most newsletters are privately owned, their revenues and costs generally remain confidential. In addition, most letters are mailed first class, so publishers are not required to release their circulation figures. For these reasons, it is difficult to obtain accurate information on the size of the industry. However, it is estimated that TSM newsletters had revenues of $34 million in 1979, and $48 million in 1982.

Number of Newsletters

The fourth edition of *The Newsletter Yearbook Directory* lists 420 newsletters that can be classified as technical, scientific or medical (see Table 5.1), a small portion of the 5000 newsletters KIPI estimated were in existence in 1981.[1] The table indicates that 156 letters, or 37.1% of the TSM letters listed in the *Directory*, are in health or health-related fields; 103, or 24.5%, are concerned with energy; and only 42, or 10%, are concerned with pure science and technology.

Table 5.1 Number of U.S. Technical, Scientific and Medical Newsletters Listed in *The Newsletter Yearbook Directory*, by Subject Category, 1983[1]

Subject	Number
Chemical/Plastics	16
Drugs/Pharmaceuticals	16
Electrical & Electronics	18
Energy/Atomic/Oil/Gas/Coal/Solar	103
Environment/Ecology	45
Health/Medicine/Hospitals/Nursing/Dental/Veterinary	136
Machinery/Manufacturing/Industrial Equipment/Engineering[2]	12
Marine/Oceanography	13
Metals & Mining/Geology	15
Psychology/Psychiatry/Mental Health	4
Science/Research & Development/Technology	42
Total	420

[1]Note: In many of these categories, the majority of the letters are directed toward management or marketing personnel rather than persons actually engaged in technical, scientific or medical activities.
[2]Only one newsletter in this category appears to be concerned with engineering.
Source: Compiled by Knowledge Industry Publications, Inc. from data in *The Newsletter Yearbook Directory, Fourth Edition*, The Newsletter Clearinghouse, 1983.

The actual number of TSM letters currently published for doctors and other health professionals, scientists and engineers is probably between

---

[1] *The Business Information Markets, 1982-1987,* Knowledge Industry Publications, Inc., White Plains, NY, 1982.

270 and 300, however. Rather than being newsletters directed to personnel actively engaged in TSM fields, many of the publications listed in the *Directory* are organization newsletters directed to their members, such as the *Chicago Herpetological Society Newsletter*, published by the Chicago Herpetological Society; letters intended for laymen with an interest in a particular field, such as the *Executive Fitness Newsletter*, published by Rodale Press, Inc.; or letters dealing with the marketing, management or regulatory aspects of a field, such as *Metals Week* and *Platt's Oilgram Price Report*, published by McGraw-Hill Publications Co., and *F-D-C Reports—"The Pink Sheet,"* published by F-D-C Reports, Inc. The *Directory*, on the other hand, does not claim to be a complete listing of all TSM letters, so the above estimate also allows for some undercounting.

An industry observer has pointed out that most newsletters in the TSM category are directed to businessmen and are not really intended for health professionals, scientists or engineers, who obtain most of their information from magazines and journals. For example, Business Publishers, Inc., publishes 29 letters, including *Energy & Minerals Resources* and *Solar Energy Intelligence Report*; however, its letters are regulatory in nature, rather than scientific or technical, and are read primarily by management personnel. A scientist would read them only to learn about new regulations (e.g., the percent of a pollutant permitted to enter the air). Similarly, the letters published by F-D-C Reports, Inc., which include titles such as *Drug Research Reports—"The Blue Sheet"* and *Medical Devices, Diagnostics and Instrumentation—"The Gray Sheet,"* contain regulatory and business information aimed at management lawyers and regulators in the health industries.

The study at hand, however, defines TSM letters as those letters intended for physicians and other health professionals, scientists and engineers. Most of these are directed to physicians; there are few letters intended for scientists and even fewer specifically for engineers. Frank Maga & Associates, in fact, although primarily an engineering firm, began publishing the *Newsletter of Engineering Analysis Software* mainly because of the lack of letters directed to engineers.

Newsletter Circulation

Newsletters in the TSM category have circulations ranging from several hundred copies to a high of 135,000 copies for *The Medical Letter*; the majority, however, have circulations of less than 5000 copies. One survey of the entire newsletter industry showed that among those with paid circulation, 42%, or nearly one-half, had less than 1001 subscribers; and 64%, or nearly two-thirds of reporting newsletters, had a circulation of less than 2001. On the basis of this information, then, and with the assumption that newsletters in the TSM category have circulation patterns similar to those in other areas, a conservative estimate of the 1983 circulation of TSM letters would be about 600,000.

Structure of the Industry

Because of the ease with which the newsletter industry may be entered, TSM newsletters range from those written and produced by one individual in a basement office to those that are part of a group of letters produced by one of the country's largest publishing houses. The majority of letters, however, are published by independent entrepreneurs. Because many newsletter publishers are privately owned, and therefore are not required to release their sales and earnings figures, and because many large publishers do not break out their newsletter revenues separately, it is impossible to make an accurate determination of the leading TSM newsletter publishers in terms of dollar sales.

However, in 1980 The Medical Letter, McGraw-Hill Publications Co. and M.J. Powers & Co. were among the largest publishers of TSM newsletters in terms of revenue. Table 5.2 presents the estimated newsletter revenue for each of them, as well as the number of TSM letters they published. Technical Insights, Inc., American Health Consultants, Inc., and The Laux Co. were among the many middle-sized publishers. (It should be noted that the largest publishers and most of the medium-sized publishers are in the medical field rather than the scientific or technical categories.)

Table 5.2 Leading TSM Newsletter Publishers, 1980

Publisher	Number of Newsletters	Estimated Newsletter Revenue, 1980 (in thousands)
The Medical Letter	1	$3,000
McGraw-Hill Publications Co.[1]	7	1,250
M.J. Powers & Co.[2]	3	950

[1]Washington Health Letter Group; in 1983 there were five letters in this group.
[2]The M.J. Powers Co., a closely held private enterprise, only releases the most general type of information about its business practices. Therefore, although represented in this table, the company is not discussed within the text that follows. In 1983 it published two newsletters.
Source: Knowledge Industry Publications, Inc.

LEADING NEWSLETTER PUBLISHERS

Because newsletters in the TSM sector cover so many different subjects, this section will describe the operations of several leading publishers, each with letters directed to a different audience.

The Medical Letter

The Medical Letter, a four-page bi-weekly costing $24.50 a year and having a circulation of 165,000, is the largest letter in the medical field, and is read by physicians, medical students, pharmaceutical manufacturers, etc. This newsletter, which was first published in 1959, is the only publication of a nonprofit independent corporation. The letter evaluates both new drugs and groups of drugs and claims to be the only source of data on drugs that is unrelated to the pharmaceutical industry.

The Medical Letter has four foreign-language editions which are printed in Spain, Japan, Switzerland (French) and Italy on a royalty basis. The French edition is also distributed in Belgium, France and Canada. The editorial content of these editions is nearly identical to that of the U.S. edition. The publication is also involved in a Continuing Medical Education program with the School of Medicine at Yale University whereby subscribers may earn credits for reading the letter and being tested on their knowledge.

Revenue of *The Medical Letter* for 1980 was estimated at $3 million.

McGraw-Hill Publications Co.

McGraw-Hill's Washington Health Letter Group is composed of five newsletters: *Long-Term Care, McGraw-Hill's Medical Utilization Review, Washington Health Record, Washington Report on Health Legislation,* and *Washington Report on Medicine and Health.* These letters are concerned with regulatory and socioeconomic information and are addressed to anyone interested in knowing the effect of government policy on the health professions: doctors, hospital and nursing home administrators, etc. (Although these letters are concerned with regulatory information, they are considered TSM letters as defined in this report because they are directed to an audience which includes health professionals rather than to an audience largely composed of management, marketing and legal personnel.)

At $367 a year, the most expensive of the Group's letters is *Washington Report on Health Legislation*. Its weekly pages deal with developments in health legislation and explain every new health-related bill. *Washington*

Report on Medicine and Health, on the other hand, is intended for readers who wish to obtain an overall view of the health field at a cost of $257 per year. Revenues of the Washington Health Letter Group were estimated at $1.25 million in 1980.

The Laux Company

Of the six letters published by The Laux Co., five are in the medical field: *Collected Letters in Surgery, Collected Letters of the International Correspondence Society of Optometrists, Infectious Disease Practice, Money Management for Physicians* and *OB-GYN Collected Letters.*

These letters all fall within the low-priced, high-circulation group with prices under $60 and circulations of 1000 copies or more.

Each of the three newsletters in the Collected Letters group resembles an advisory service for a particular specialty. A physician will write seeking advice on the treatment of a problem patient; this letter is then sent to a panel of experts who attempt to answer the query. Both the letter and its reply are subsequently printed in the newsletter.

Money Management for Physicians and *Collected Letters of the International Correspondence Society of Optometrists* are sponsored publications, and in this respect they differ from most other newsletters. Several advertisers each purchase a portion of *Money Management's* circulation. The editorial content remains the same throughout the issue, but each advertiser receives a four-page insert in its segment of the circulation. (*Collected Letters of the International Correspondence Society of Optometrists* is sponsored by a single advertiser who receives an advertising insert in the entire circulation of the issue.) The newsletter is then mailed to recipients selected by the advertiser and to some paid subscribers as well.

Technical Insights, Inc.

Technical Insights publishes four newsletters: *Inside R&D, Biomass Digest, Industrial Robots International* and *Genetic Technology News.* These letters, which contain both scientific and policy information, are read by upper-level research managers who have broad responsibilities for new technology. About 25% of their circulation is outside the United States.

Inside R&D, a weekly, is aimed at research and development managers and deals with new technical developments and policies. It has several thousand readers throughout the world and is priced at $252 a year. *Biomass Digest* is a newsletter concerned with the use of green plants to produce energy (gasohol or fire) and chemicals. It was launched in 1979 and costs

$168 per year. *Industrial Robots International* was started in 1980 and costs $192 per year; and *Genetic Technology News* was begun in 1981 and costs $180.

In addition to covering new technical developments and policies, the latter three letters are also information services. They abstract important technical papers, list new patents and grants when they are issued, carry a bibliography of significant journal articles and list important meetings in their fields. The company's newsletter revenue in 1980 was estimated at $540,000, or 75% of total revenue.

American Health Consultants

This company publishes 12 monthly letters in health-related areas, ranging in price from $78 to $168.

The letters, with titles such as *Employee Health & Fitness, Hospital Admitting Monthly, Hospital Employee Health* and *Prospective Payment Survival*, are generally directed to hospital committees, hospital administrators and others concerned with hospital operations, although a few, such as *Back Pain Monitor* and *Contraceptive Technology Update*, are directed to health professionals in specific fields. In late 1983 the company announced an agreement with Mead Data Central to include the full text of its letters in a planned online medical information research service.

Quest Publishing Co.

Quest Publishing Co. publishes four letters in the field of medical technology: *Biomedical Safety and Standards, Biomedical Technology Information Service, Clinical Lab Letter* and *Radiology Letter*. These letters, all of which emphasize the technological aspects of the field more than the medical, contain data on new hospital technology, hazardous products and recalls, government regulations, and safety and standards. They are read by hospital administrators and directors, engineers and technologists in hospitals, and manufacturers of technology for hospitals. Subscription rates range from $92 for *Biomedical Safety and Standards*, which has an estimated circulation of 2500, to $120 for *Clinical Lab Letter* and *Radiology Letter*. Although Quest also publishes the *Journal of Clinical Engineering* and an annual, newsletters are its largest source of sales and profits.

Competition

It should be noted that most of the above newsletter publishers feel that they have no head-to-head competition in their area of expertise. In the majority of cases, their letters cover an aspect of the TSM Field untouched by any other publisher except, perhaps, in a peripheral manner, and there is little overlap of information. Thus, a subscription to one of these publications is important to a professional who wishes the latest data in his or her field.

ECONOMICS OF NEWSLETTER PUBLISHING

Starting a Newsletter

To be successful, a newsletter must aim at a clearly defined niche in the market and its potential readers must understand the significance of the field it covers. It should contain a large amount of proprietary information that the reader knows will be unavailable elsewhere for a period of time or, failing this, it must add value to the information it contains in the form of analysis, interpretation or authoritative opinion.

The size of the potential market must be large enough to support the letter but not so large that the letter lacks a clear focus or unique information. Newsletters seem to do best in fields that are changing rapidly and in which there is a tremendous need to keep up.

The number of letters already serving the market should also be investigated, along with the market's willingness and ability to pay for the letter. The latter point is important because the potential universe of a letter will vary with its price; there is one universe at $2000 and quite another at $20. A few years ago consultant Paul J. Bringe listed five market conditions that can make for a successful newsletter operation; they are still true today:

•The market is broad and served by many periodicals, but with too much lag between writing and publishing.

•The market is narrow with few or no periodicals serving it.

•The market is professional or semiprofessional requiring information not generally available elsewhere.

•The market is fast-moving, with last week's or last month's information largely obsolete today.

•The market is highly specialized, with intense interest in a subject existing within a relatively small group.

All these conditions exist to varying degrees within the TSM market.

How Much Capital is Necessary?

In theory, newsletters are relatively inexpensive to start. Article after article states that all an entrepreneur needs is a desk, a typewriter and $10,000 for start-up costs to cover initial promotion. However, many observers of the TSM newsletter field feel it is impossible to launch a letter today for much less than $60,000. If it is started for less money, the entrepreneur is probably not spending enough on promotion and, as a result, is not getting an accurate idea of the potential for the letter.

The actual amount of capital required to launch a letter depends a great deal on the kind of publication involved. A high-circulation, low-priced letter usually requires more initial capital than a low-circulation, high-priced letter because of the need for a greater number of mailings in order to gain a large number of subscribers.

Starting costs also depend on whether the would-be publisher already has existing letters in allied fields. For example, *Weather and Climate Report,* published by Nautilus Press, Inc., serves the same constituency as its *Ocean Science News,* and many of their subscribers are identical. It was promoted to *Ocean Science News* subscribers in the same envelope as the newsletter. Thus, at no extra mailing cost this promotion reached a group of prospective readers already familiar with the publisher's product.

How Long Before Break-even?

The length of time it takes for a newsletter to break even depends on the type of letter, the size of the potential market, how "hot" the subject is and the speed with which the letter acquires subscribers.

One industry analyst points out that there are two broad classes of letters: those that are priced at $100 or more and should break even in the first year; and low-priced, high-circulation letters that may take two to three years to break even. Many TSM publishers, however, believe that a new letter should break even in the first year, regardless of price. (Publishers in this category tend to be producers of several letters, a factor that may make a break-even status easier to attain from an accounting viewpoint.) Others in the industry expect a newsletter to take from two to five years to break even, though a publisher should know whether a letter will succeed by the results of its mailings in the first six months.

Reasons for Failure

Although the newsletter market is relatively easy to enter, many letters fail to become successful. Reasons for failure can include competition from existing letters on the same or similar subjects, ineffective renewal techniques and inability to include essential information. Failure may also result if the subject is a fad, the letter is aimed at too broad an audience, competition exists from other channels of information or readership is difficult to define. (A publisher must be able to define its readers and know where to reach them.)

Subscription Acquisition

Generally, newsletter subscriptions are obtained by direct mail promotions, which may include a sample copy, a trial subscription offer, or a premium such as a special report. Nautilus Press, publisher of several letters on oceanography, has acquired subscriptions mainly through its exhibits at meetings in the field. Other publishers use telephone selling as their primary method of generating new subscriptions.

The amount of money spent to acquire a subscription varies and depends to a great extent on the success of the promotion. One publisher claims that the average newsletter subscriber will continue his subscription for seven years; therefore, one subscriber will bring in revenue equal to seven times the annual subscription rate. The publisher must decide how much of this revenue it is willing to spend initially to acquire the subscription. Another publisher states that a mailing should not only offset its costs but should also return a substantial increment above costs. Most established publishers are willing to spend the first year's revenue in order to acquire a new subscription. Once a subscriber is acquired, a publisher can make money not only on that subscriber's renewal but also on that person's purchase of its other newsletters and products.

Renewal Rates

Generally, the more specialized the newsletter, the higher the renewal rate; in addition, a more mature publication tends to have a higher renewal rate than a newer one. The lowest renewal rate occurs in the first year when many fringe subscribers fail to renew because the letter does not meet their expectations.

Many industry analysts say that the minimum renewal rate after the first year should be more than 50%, with the percentage increasing annually; if a renewal rate is 50% or less, it may be a signal that the editorial product needs improvement. After the first year, the renewal rate should rise to 70% or 80%, and many successful letters have a renewal rate of 75% to 90%. The higher the renewal rate, the lower the marketing expenses required to obtain renewals and expand circulation. Some experts, however, feel that renewal rates in the high 80%s or better may indicate that a letter has not fully tapped its potential. Renewal rates in the TSM newsletter field are generally well over 70% with many in the high 80%s or low 90%s. This could be an indication that the industry is not reaching its full potential readership.

Circulation Growth

Generally, a newsletter experiences a period of rapid growth for two or three years, followed by increasing subscription acquisition costs and a leveling-off of circulation. If a publisher is dissatisfied with this situation, it can create another letter (perhaps on a different facet of the same topic), offer its services as a consultant or market related products, such as directories, reports or seminars, to the subscribers.

Pricing

A newsletter publisher must have the right combination of price, product and market. In theory, a publisher must price in such a way as to maximize gross dollar income (not circulation) while minimizing costs; that is, the publisher must price its product to yield the greatest long-term dollar income from subscription and collateral sales at the lowest cost. If additional circulation is too expensive to acquire, a newsletter is better off without it. Few publishers can afford elaborate price testing. Instead they follow traditional price lines, use intuition or common sense and watch what other publishers are doing.

Resistance to the price of a newsletter is usually related to customs in the field, the subscriber's ability to pay and competition from other letters, journals or magazines. For example, *Infectious Disease Practice*, published by The Laux Co. and having an estimated circulation of 2000 at a price of $57, has experienced some price resistance. The publisher assumed that potential subscribers compared the price to such publications as *The Medical Letter* ($24.50) and the *New England Journal of Medicine* ($48). Price resistance also reflects prospective subscribers' failure to understand that advertising pays all or most of the costs of magazines, while a newsletter relies solely on subscription revenue.

In the newsletter field as a whole, low-priced, high-circulation letters are in the minority: most letters have prices starting above $70 and rising to several thousand dollars. McGraw-Hill's *Washington Report on Health Legislation*, priced at $367, and International Bio-Medical Information Service's *Bio-Medical Insight*, which is $350, are among the most expensive letters in the TSM field. Both these letters have estimated circulations of 1000 to 2000, so although they are high-priced, their circulations are not low, except perhaps in a relative sense. *The Medical Letter,* on the other hand, with a price of $24.50, has a circulation of 135,000; and M.J. Powers & Co.'s *Nurses' Drug Alert*, priced at $22, has an estimated circulation of over 50,000.

There are exceptions, also, to the rule that specialized newsletters are generally high-priced, low-circulation letters. *Collected Letters in Surgery*, addressed to surgeons, and *OB-GYN Collected Letters,* directed to obstetricians and gynecologists, both published by The Laux Co., with estimated circulations of over 1000, are priced at $57 and $54, respectively.

The major advantage of a mass market or high-circulation letter at a low price is the size of its subscriber list, which provides opportunities for the sale of various other products. A letter with a limited market, on the other hand, has lower production and fulfillment costs and, because it has a relatively small number of subscribers, is better able to secure renewals through personal contact.

In addition, a high-priced, low-circulation newsletter seems to have more price elasticity than a low-priced letter. High-priced letters rarely encounter resistance to a price increase, presumably because of the need for the specialized information they provide. When the price of a low-priced letter is raised even by a slight amount, on the other hand, the renewal rate will generally decline. The degree of price elasticity of a newsletter may depend more on its subject matter than on its price, however. The Laux Co., for example, purchased *OB-GYN Collected Letters* in 1976 when its subscription price was $28. It subsequently boosted the price to $54 in several steps while keeping circulation stable and maintaining a high renewal rate.

Because of the growth of available information in the TSM field, it is likely that the proportion of high-priced, low-circulation letters will increase in the future.

Economics of Multiple Newsletters

Many publishers in the TSM field produce several newsletters. McGraw-Hill, for example, publishes five letters in the health field; Technical Insights publishes five letters in the sci-tech area and Nautilus Press publishes four letters on oceanography and meteorology. Publishers of multiple letters sometimes achieve minor economies in paper and printing, and may also accommodate an additional newsletter with no increase in facilities or editorial staff; thus spreading fixed costs over a larger revenue base. In some instances, the same information can be used for articles in more than one newsletter, resulting in further editorial economies. For example, M.J. Powers & Co. publishes two letters—*Nurses' Drug Alert* and *Physicians' Drug Alert*—addressed to nurses and doctors. Each letter reports on recent occurrences of adverse drug reactions and drug interactions. Although the original information is identical, the material is written differently for each letter.

Also, less promotion may be necessary in order to persuade subscribers to one letter to purchase another and, if circulation levels off, subscribers can be swung to another existing letter or to a completely new one. Finally, with multiple letters it is easier for a publisher to sell its other products to subscribers.

Revenue and Expense Model

Table 5.3 is a model of the revenue and expense involved in the marketing of a weekly newsletter priced at $175 per year. The sensitivity of newsletters both to the size of their circulation and to renewal rates is illustrated by depicting the letter's profit and loss at varying levels of circulation renewal.

Editorial expense, the largest cost, remains fixed over the range of circulations shown in the table. Fulfillment expense, the main variable cost, is only slightly sensitive to volume. In the model, the cost of printing and mailing an issue of the letter is about 55 cents at a circulation of 300, declining to about 45 cents at a circulation of 1000—hardly a significant amount in total dollar terms. Marketing cost is extremely sensitive both to renewal rates and to market size. In the model, the difference between renewal rates of 80% and 60% is a doubling of marketing costs, and these same costs more than triple as circulation rises from 300 to 1000.

INTERNATIONAL SALES

The attitude of publishers of TSM newsletters toward international marketing of their products varies. Several publishers say they do not actively solicit foreign subscriptions; however, if foreign names are on their mailing lists, they will be solicited. Although some extra costs can be recouped by adding a surcharge for foreign subscribers, some publishers note that the international airmail rate of 40 cents per half-ounce results in sizable costs for invoicing, mailing and renewal promotions of international subscriptions. Some publishers, however, do find it profitable to promote their letters overseas.

Table 5.3 Revenue and Expenses for a Weekly Newsletter Priced at $175 Annually, by Circulation and Renewal Rates[1]

	Circulation					
	300		500		1000	
Renewal rate	60%	80%	60%	80%	60%	80%
Revenues	$52,500	$52,500	$87,500	$87,500	$175,000	$175,000
Expenses						
Editorial	60,000	60,000	60,000	60,000	60,000	60,000
Fulfillment	9,000	9,000	13,000	13,000	23,500	23,500
Marketing	10,200	5,100	17,000	8,500	34,000	17,000
Operating profit (loss)	($26,700)	($21,600)	($ 2,500)	$ 6,000	$ 57,500	$ 74,500

[1] Assumes 0.3% return on new mailings; cost of acquiring a new subscription is $85.
Source: Knowledge Industry Publications, Inc.

EXPANDING THE REVENUE BASE

Newsletter operation affords an opportunity for substantial supplementary income. Subscribers develop a loyalty to a publication and form a customer base through which related materials can be sold. It is also true that these additional products may introduce nonsubscriber purchasers to the parent publication. The materials may be spin-offs from the newsletter itself or new services or products that use existing customer lists. Spin-offs are highly profitable because the research has already been done for the parent publication, which results in relatively low "people costs."

Following are examples of some of the revenue-expanding activities of several publishers.

Technical Insights publishes a series of reports on emerging technologies, covering topics such as nitrogen fixation, heat storage and industrial robots. These reports, each about 200 pages long, are concerned with technology rather than marketing, and range in price from $200 to $520.

American Health Consultants sponsored seven national conferences on health-related topics in 1983. The company also recently signed a contract with Mead Data Central to include the full text of its newsletters in Mead's forthcoming online medical information research service.

Quest Publishing issues *Guide to Biomedical Standards,* an annual listing of worldwide standards. Subscribers to its newsletter, *Biomedical Safety and Standards,* receive the directory at no charge; nonsubscribers can purchase it for $12.

The Laux Co. offers annual bound volumes of *Collected Letters in Surgery* and *OB-GYN Collected Letters* for $18.95 each.

As was previously mentioned, *The Medical Letter* licenses four foreign-language editions which are printed in Spain, Japan, Switzerland (French) and Italy on a royalty basis.

Newsletter publishers also rent out their mailing lists and sell back issues and reprints of their letters.

It should be noted that sometimes a publisher in another field will develop a newsletter as a means of recycling information and expanding its revenue base. Year Book Medical Publishers, for example, publishes *The Year Book of Pediatrics Newsletter* and *The Year Book of Urology Newsletter*, both of which inform physicians of new developments in their fields that have been reported in various journal articles (with a citation).

ECRI (formerly the Emergency Care Research Institute) publishes six newsletters in its Technology for Health Care series. Each is directed to a specific hospital department, such as emergency medicine, anesthesiology, cardiology, respiratory therapy, surgery and materials management. The first title purchased costs $60 for members and $70 for nonmembers; prices of additional letters are on a sliding scale with a top for all six letters of $290 for members and $335 for nonmembers. ECRI, which claims to be the world's leading independent organization dedicated to health-care technology, facilities and procedures, was probably the earliest publisher in the field of medical technology. Its publications evaluate medical technology, describe problem areas and alert users to hazardous equipment; however, these publications are costly and are mainly purchased by health-care institutions. The series described above was initiated by ECRI in order to republish data for physicians and allied health professionals at low cost.

INDUSTRY PROBLEMS

The newsletter industry today is faced with several problems: these include rising costs, increased competition from other letters on the same subject, photocopying and the high cost of postage combined with poor postal service.

Photocopying

Despite the fact that it is illegal under the copyright laws, photocopying of newsletters remains an industry problem. There is little that can be done to enforce the laws, nor have publishers found any paper or ink that cannot be reproduced. Some publishers attempt to combat photocopying by offering a discount for multiple subscriptions.

Photocopying is probably less of a problem in the sci-tech field than in many other areas. Scientists and engineers constantly deal with information, are aware of the issue of copyright violation and are prone to pay for what they read. In many instances, also, the letters are relatively inexpensive, resulting in the willing purchase of several copies.

Postage and Poor Postal Service

The high cost of postage coupled with poor postal service is one of the major problems of an industry that depends on prompt delivery. High postage rates not only affect the cost of mailing the letter itself but also increase billing and promotion costs. In addition, poor postal delivery often erodes the timeliness of the information the letter may contain.

THE FUTURE

As long as readers are willing and able to pay their subscription prices, newsletters have good prospects for the future. It is difficult and expensive for professionals to keep track of the TSM information related to their fields of interest and, in addition, to sort out the important from the insignificant. If newsletters perform this task well, they will continue to be successful.

The medical area is filling rapidly with newsletters and is becoming quite competitive. Hence, a shakeout of certain publications is possible. The number of newsletters is also increasing in the sci-tech area, and should continue to keep pace with the flow of information in this sector. Moreover, large publishers of other forms of scientific information are beginning to recognize the opportunities present in the newsletter field.

In considering the future of TSM newsletters it should be remembered that a newsletter is simply a means of delivering information, and the medium through which this information is delivered is purely incidental. Many technological advances in the ability to communicate information will probably occur within the next five or 10 years. Even now, through vendors such as NewsNet, newsletters may be sent electronically from the publisher directly to a subscriber's desktop terminal. It is extremely unlikely, however, that electronic newsletters will replace print in the foreseeable future. Electronic letters lack the convenient portability of the print version nor is a terminal as easy to read from as "old-fashioned" print.

LOOSE-LEAF SERVICES

Loose-leaf services are a rare commodity in the TSM field. Few services exist in the sci-tech area. In 1981 Hemisphere Publishing Corp. began publishing the *Heat Exchanger Design Handbook*, a loose-leaf engineering handbook that is updated twice a year; it is the only service available to the public in the engineering field. There are only a small number of companies publishing in the medical sector, although several services, such as those published by Aspen Systems Corp., exist in the health-law or hospital-management field. Total revenues of TSM loose-leaf services were estimated at $6 million in 1982.

Harper & Row is the major publisher of loose-leaf services in the medical field. Its 10 medical and dental services are similar in format to those in the business field; they consist of a binder or binders containing basic material on a given subject supplemented by periodic updatings. (Through a subsidiary, Facts & Comparisons, Inc., Harper also publishes two looseleaf services—*Facts and Comparisons (Drug Information Compendium)*, which provides current data on over 10,000 drug products, and *Drug Interaction Facts,* which provides information on drug interactions.)

The services are multi-authored, multivolume reference sets covering various medical specialties. Each set offers comprehensive coverage of one area of medicine, such as dermatology, otolaryngology or pediatrics, with continuous updating provided by an annual revision service.

The loose-leaf services are kept up-to-date by annually substituting "new pages for old." Each year subscribers to the revision service receive a set of new pages, which includes revised information to be substituted for out-of-date material, additions to existing chapters and totally new chapters when these are necessary. A complete new index is also prepared annually in order to provide an instant cross-reference for all subjects. Because of each service's loose-leaf format, inserting and removing pages is not a problem.

Each service contains specific clinical information on the state of the art, including diagnosis and therapy. They are meant to be comprehensive reference sources and the revision process means they can be more up-to-date than a textbook, which is a year or more behind the field on publication date.

Inherent in a loose-leaf service, also, is a flexibility that is lacking in a bound book. If a book has 82 contributors, for example, its publisher must hold its publication until all the material is in; with a loose-leaf service, certain contributions can be sent as part of the next update. Loose-leaf services are also revised occasionally, rather than simply being updated. Harper's six-volume *Gynecology and Obstetrics*, for example, underwent a revision in recent years because changes in the specialty had made it obsolete.

Speed

Unlike loose-leaf services in the business field where speed is important both in the introduction of a new service and in the dissemination of information to subscribers to an existing service, speed is relatively unimportant to a medical service. When a new medical discovery is made, it may have side effects and drawbacks that take some time to appear. The academicians who write the services generally have a conservative approach and wait for these problems to surface. Thus, a medical service must be current but should not be in the forefront of the field.

Amount of Material

Each of Harper's services is composed of from three to 12 volumes, and each volume contains 700 to 1000 pages. The number of volumes in a service varies depending on the specialty—*Clinical Medicine* has 12 volumes, while *Biomedical Foundations of Ophthalmology* has three volumes. The amount of material distributed has increased over the years, and new volumes are sometimes added when the contents are updated. Harper aims for a minimum of 10% of new pages each year.

Subscription Rates

Harper's loose-leaf services are sold at prices ranging from $300 for the three-volume *Biomedical Foundations of Ophthalmology* to $600 for the 12-volume *Clinical Medicine*. Rates for the annual revision services range from $25 for *Biomedical Foundations of Ophthalmology* to $75 for *Clinical Medicine*.

Leading Companies

Harper & Row is by far the major company in the TSM loose-leaf service field with estimated annual sales in 1980 of $4 million. Other important publishers in the field are Scientific American and Futura Press.

In 1978, Scientific American began publishing *Scientific American Medicine*, a 2000-page, two-volume service that provides the physician with current information on patient problems he or she is likely to encounter in daily practice. Each month subscribers to the service receive an update package containing current information on various subjects and a new index. The initial subscription price for this service is $235, which includes the two volumes, binders and monthly updates. Subscribers may also enroll, at no additional charge, in a continuing medical education program based on the contents of *Scientific American Medicine* and sponsored by the School of Medicine at Stanford University.

Futura Press has published six volumes of *Modern Technics In Surgery*, a projected 10-volume series on current operative procedures. It hopes to publish two more volumes in 1984. Initial volumes cost $49.50 each; new installments, issued at least once a year, are an average of $35 each.

Economics of Loose-Leaf Service Publishing

Subscription Acquisition and Renewal

Although medical loose-leaf services are intended for physicians already in practice, their major sales thrust is aimed at residents in the hope that they will continue to subscribe throughout their careers. Libraries also purchase the services. More than two-thirds of the sales of Harper's services are through salesmen; the remaining portion of sales are through direct mail and convention exhibits. Harper does not lose money in acquiring a subscription, but it spends a great deal to obtain it. Renewals of the initial subscription, however, are obtained by mail at relatively low cost. Thus, the major portion of a service's profit comes from renewals.

Renewal rates for the services average about 90%; normally a subscription is canceled only at a physician's retirement or death. Therefore, when a subscriber purchases a service, the publisher is virtually assured of renewal income for many years.

New Services

A new service is introduced when the publisher feels the market will support it and competent editors are available to staff it. It is introduced as quickly as possible but usually it takes a few years to issue all the sections in the service. For example, Harper's *Clinical Medicine*, in 12 volumes, was published in a three-year program. Normally, it costs upwards of $250,000 to $500,000 to launch a new service, depending on its size. Thus, there is a sizable risk involved in establishing a new service because of the large initial investment that is required.

If a service is successful, it will generally be two to three years before it shows a profit. It will peak fairly quickly in terms of subscription sales, however, and will then gain subscriptions more slowly.

FUTURE OF LOOSE-LEAF SERVICES

Growth in the loose-leaf service area can occur in several ways: price increases; growth in the circulation of established services; introduction of new services serving new markets; and the addition of new or related activities.

That price increases will expand the revenue base is fairly obvious. It should be remembered, however, that most price increases are used to pass along real increases in costs: reporting on new developments in a field can involve amended pages, indexes and, sometimes, completely new chapters, on a regular basis.

Since the market for existing services is relatively stable, it is unlikely that a publication will see a major surge in circulation. Introducing a new service can enable a smaller company to expand its revenue base, though it has less effect on a large publisher. To gain $1 million in revenue from a new publication with a subscription price of $200, for example, would require 5000 subscribers—quite a high number.

Recycling information or launching new ventures related in some way to existing publications can be an important means of increasing the revenue of a loose-leaf service publisher. A publisher may select a section; add a title page, table of contents and index; and bind it for sale to a peripheral market that is not reached by the service itself. For example, "Introduction to Neuroradiology," a chapter in Harper's *Clinical Neurology*, has been bound separately and marketed to radiologists. Similarly, its *Clinical Ophthalmology* service contains a chapter on neuro-ophthalmology which has been bound separately and marketed to neurologists. In each case, prospective purchasers are informed of the source of the material.

Other opportunities for related activities include the sponsoring of seminars and conferences and the publication of newsletters related to the subjects of the loose-leaf services.

Outlook

As the number of persons involved in technical, scientific or medical professions increases and the volume of knowledge in these sectors increases, the demand for loose-leaf services will also increase. Although there are currently only a few loose-leaf publishers in the medical field and few in the sci-tech area, the outlook is favorable both for the growth of existing publishers and for the appearance of new ones. It would seem that an organized body of data, updated periodically, in specialized areas within each field should be able to find a market as a current reference source.

6

Database Publishing: Print and Online

This book will define a database as an organized collection of data, usually in machine-readable form. A database publisher assembles and disseminates such information in a variety of formats. In order to be considered a database, however, a product must have several key characteristics, among them comprehensiveness, in-depth indexing and ease of retrieval of specific items. In addition, a database product is intended for reference use rather than for casual reading.

A database may be in printed form (hard copy) or computerized (online). Many print databases are simply regularly issued bulletins of abstracts of the literature on a given subject. Computer-based or online services are a result of the ever-increasing avalanche of scientific and technical (sci-tech) literature and the increased costs of acquiring it. The sheer volume of data and the need to update and analyze the databank at regular intervals made it nearly impossible to rely solely on manual systems and get the job done. Therefore, publishers of conventional abstracting and indexing services switched to photocomposition and other computer-aided production techniques, and they found that extensive files of machine-readable bibliographic data emerged as a by-product. From there it was a short step to supplement their print product lines with magnetic tapes containing much the same information for search and retrieval by computer.

The primary difference between hard-copy and computerized databases, therefore, is in their final format. If the data are regularly published in a print format, they comprise a print database. If the customer has direct access to the computerized database via a terminal, the database is termed online. (It should be noted, however, that nearly all online databases are also available in print.)

Online databases enable a user to rapidly retrieve specific information from a vast collection of stored data. They are of two types: bibliographic and nonbibliographic. A bibliographic database usually includes a bibliographic citation plus an abstract of the cited material, which may be a book, article, report, patent, etc. In some cases, however, this type of database includes only the citation and the access numbers of the cited documents; in a growing number of instances, it includes the full text of the material. Examples of bibliographic databases include CA SEARCH, an online version of *Chemical Abstracts* and the CLAIMS™ series of patent databases published by IFI/Plenum Data Co., a division of Plenum Publishing Corp. Nonbibliographic databases are of two types: textual and numeric. Textual databases may contain organization names and addresses, legal decisions, newspaper articles, transportation routes, technologies available for license, etc.; Control Data's Technotec database is an example of this type. Numeric databases generally contain descriptive and/or engineering data on various industries, materials, drugs, etc.; many numeric databases come with programs that permit the data to be manipulated in order to perform various kinds of analyses.

Databases can also be categorized as source databases or reference databases. Source databases contain original or "source" information and directly provide answers or estimates. They are primarily numeric, but also include full-text and chemical/physical properties databases, such as those produced by Chemical Abstracts Service. Reference databases contain references to the original information to guide a user to its source; they include bibliographic databases with or without the abstract of the original material.

The online database business originated with sci-tech databases; each of these generally covers a particular branch of science or technology and consists of bibliographic files of citations and abstracts of scientific journal articles, research reports, conference proceedings, monographs, etc. Most sci-tech databases were originally compiled by not-for-profit organizations and government agencies. They were computerized to expedite print publication as well as to lower search costs and improve efficiency. The databases were then made commercially available to help cover costs and to broaden use. With the development of online access, their use increased rapidly and commercial publishers entered the field.

SIZE AND STRUCTURE OF THE DATABASE INDUSTRY

The market for hard-copy and online technical, scientific and medical

(TSM) database publishing in 1982 is estimated at $660 million, of which $125 million was online and $535 million was print. These figures include revenues of government and not-for-profit organizations, as well as revenues of database vendors. (Revenues of the business information industry, by comparison, are estimated at more than $9 billion.)

No exact figures are available on the number of companies involved in TSM database publishing. According to the Information Industry Association (IIA), in 1982 there were 1249 U.S.-based companies in the business of supplying information; this figure excludes, by definition, not-for-profit organizations and government agencies, among others. IIA figures indicate that there were 324 for-profit companies involved in TSM database publishing in 1982. The addition of not-for-profit organizations engaged in TSM database publishing probably raises the total number of companies to about 400.

The total number of computer-readable databases and records contained in databases has greatly increased over the past several years. In early 1984 there were an estimated 175 bibliographic, textual or full-text databases in the TSM area produced in the United States. From 1957 to 1983 the number of unique items covered by full voting members and associate members of the National Federation of Abstracting and Information Services increased from 443,702 in 1957 to over 3.6 million in 1983, a 718.3% increase (see Table 6.1).

The number of online database searches conducted via the major U.S. and Canadian bibliographic retrieval systems has also increased greatly during the last few years. Among the factors responsible for the dramatic increase in search volume are increased awareness of online databases on the part of potential users; improved marketing of online search services by vendors; and the growing variety of databases and their enhanced value as retrospective tools, since online files currently contain many more years of back information.

Leading Companies

Because many of the leading database producers are divisions of large commercial or not-for-profit organizations that do not break out their database revenues separately, and because privately owned firms are not required to disclose their annual sales and earnings figures, it is impossible to determine accurately the leading companies in terms of sales.

It should also be noted that due to the wide range of prices of online databases, several industry experts believe revenue to be an unfair parameter by which to determine leading companies. Revenues from the National Library of Medicine's databases are relatively small, for example,

Table 6.1 Number of Unique Items Covered by Members of National Federation of Abstracting and Information Services, Selected Years, 1957-1983

	1957	1962	1967	1972	1977	1981	1982	1983[1]
American Institute of Physics	—	—	—	30,000	21,435	24,869	26,531	28,000
BioSciences Information Service	40,061	100,858	125,026	240,006	250,148	300,000	315,000	335,000
Chemical Abstracts Service[2]	102,525	175,138	269,293	379,048	478,225	549,326	557,447	570,000
Engineering Information, Inc.	26,797	38,120	51,670	83,653	97,380	106,643	179,300	215,000
National Library of Medicine[3]	104,517	150,000	165,000	221,000	259,980	279,000	282,180	286,000
All other members and affiliates	169,802	232,941	473,680	664,736	907,422	1,911,684	2,081,279	2,196,763
Total	443,702	697,057	1,084,669	1,598,443	2,014,590	3,171,522	3,441,737	3,630,763

[1] Estimate.
[2] Statistics exclude book reviews, of which there are 3000 to 4000 citations a year.
[3] These figures include *Index Medicus* and special list citations.
Source: National Federation of Abstracting and Information Services, February 1983.

yet this organization accounts for a large portion of all online searches in the United States and Canada.

Yet, certain companies emerge as leaders in their respective sectors of the TSM field, among them Chemical Abstracts Service, a division of the American Chemical Society; the National Library of Medicine; Engineering Information, Inc. and the Institute for Scientific Information. Table 6.2 indicates 1980 revenue of these producers for both hard-copy and online TSM services. With the exception of the National Library of Medicine, online revenues were generally the smaller portion of total revenues; on the average, they accounted for about 15% of the revenue from TSM databases. The table illustrates that there is a wide range in revenues among publishers of TSM databases. Revenues of the companies listed ranged from $3 million to $36 million in 1980, for example, yet each is a leader in its particular segment of the TSM database spectrum.

Table 6.2 Revenue of Selected Database Publishers in TSM Field, 1980 (in millions)

	Revenue		
Publisher	Online	Hardcopy	Total
Chemical Abstracts Service	$4.0	$32.0	$36.0
Institute for Scientific Information	1.0	19.0	20.0
Engineering Index[1]	0.9	2.4	3.3
National Library of Medicine	2.0	1.0	3.0

[1] In 1981 Engineering Index changed its name to Engineering Information, Inc.
Sources: Knowledge Industry Publications, Inc. estimates based on information from company spokesmen.

HOW ONLINE DATABASES WORK

There are two ways to gain access to online databases and obtain the results of online searches. A company may either employ an information retailer that has access to the desired databanks, or it may purchase, rent or lease a computer terminal and obtain access itself to major online systems and databases. The latter method is the most preferred in the sci-tech field. In order to gain direct access, a potential customer must first obtain a computer terminal. Terminals can be rented or leased for as little as $85 to $150 a month or they can be purchased outright for under $2000.

Access to online systems and databases varies in cost. Many systems have no minimum or fixed charges, and vendors simply bill the customer for the search time used at prices ranging from $15 to $300 per hour and up, although the average cost is between $35 and $105. Since most searches require only 10 to 15 minutes to complete, the average cost for a completed search is generally between $5.50 and $26.50. (It should be kept in mind, however, that the "true cost" of an online search is somewhat higher, for in figuring the cost of a search, a user must also consider the fees of a trained staff member to conduct the search, overhead, and charges for data communications network services; the cost of these services through TYMNET and TELENET is $8 per hour, while the cost through UNINET is $6 per hour.)

Online databases are made available to users through information vendors; that is, organizations that publicly sell their own or other producers' databases on their computer system. Three types of organizations offer online access to databases: computer time-sharing bureaus, such as Control Data Corp., that, in addition to the remote computing facilities they offer, also make databases available for their clients to search; services dedicated exclusively to offering databases, such as DIALOG Information Services, Inc., a subsidiary of Lockheed Corp.; and database producers, such as Mead Data Central, that, in addition to producing a database, offer it exclusively on one of their own computer systems. (In the TSM field, for example, Chemical Abstracts Service offers CAS ONLINE through its own computer system, and the National Library of Medicine offers its MEDLARS database through its own system, as well as through commercial database vendors.)

To perform a search of a databank—i.e., to look for information in a database—a set of appropriate terms is entered into the computer. In a matter of seconds the computer will respond with an answer that appears either on the terminal screen or on a printout; some systems provide answers in both forms.

Dialog Information Services, Inc.

Dialog Information Services, Inc. began in 1969 with a single database. Today, with more than 180 databases, Dialog claims to be the largest system of its kind in the world, containing over 80 million records that provide references to over 60,000 worldwide publications in over 40 languages, including technical reports, conference papers, newspapers, journal and magazine articles, patents and statistical data. These databases cover subjects such as agriculture, business, chemistry, social sciences, biology and engineering; arithmetic and statistical manipulative techniques are also available. Table 6.3 lists Dialog's databases together with their online connect time charges.

Dialog's fee structure is based on computer connect time (the length of time during which the user's terminal is in communication with the computer). Ordinarily, there are no start-up, minimum or subscription fees, but there is a small charge, ranging in most instances from 10 cents to 90 cents for each citation printed and mailed to the user. There are also discounts of $5 to $15 per hour which come into effect as a customer's volume of usage increases.

Other leading database vendors in the United States include Bibliographic Retrieval Services (BRS), National Library of Medicine (NLM) and System Development Corp. (SDC).

Estimated annual revenues for Lockheed, SDC and BRS in 1980 were about $30 million, $8 million and $6 million, respectively. Since about 75% of their business involved sci-tech databases, revenues generated from this area amounted to $23 million (Lockheed), $6 million (SDC) and $4.5 million (BRS).

DESCRIPTIONS OF SELECTED DATABASE PUBLISHERS

Because there are so many different types of databases and database publishing operations, this section will describe the operations of several important database publishers, each of which serves a different segment of the TSM market.

Engineering Information, Inc.

Engineering Information, Inc. (Ei) (formerly Engineering Index) is a not-for-profit organization recognized as the leading international publisher of multidisciplinary engineering bibliographic data; it is the largest engineering database publisher in the United States. Ei's database incorporates 2.5 million abstracts representing a large variety of engineering subjects. Over 3500 journals and 2000 conference proceedings from 40 countries in 20 languages are used as primary sources, and about 9000 records are added to the database each month.

The organization's principal print products are *Engineering Index Monthly* and *Engineering Index Annual*. The *Monthly*, which costs $1290, provides current awareness of rapidly changing technological developments in science and industry by supplying up-to-date technical information on significant engineering/research developments; an average of 9000 abstracts appears in each issue. The 1983 *Annual*, a cumulation of all records published in the preceding year's monthly issues, costs $710 and contains over 100,000 abstracts.

(Text continued on page 149.)

Table 6.3 Online Databases Offered by DIALOG Information Services, Inc.[1] and Their Online Connect Time Rates, July 1983

Database (Supplier)	Online Connect Time Rate (per hour)
Chemistry	
CA SEARCH (Chemical Abstracts Service)	$68
Chemical Exposure (Chemical Effects Information Center, Oak Ridge National Laboratory)	45
Chemical Industry Notes (American Chemical Society)	74
Chemical Regulations and Guidelines System (U.S. Interagency Regulatory Liason Group, CRC Systems Inc.)	70
Chemlaw (Bureau of National Affairs, Fein-Marquart Associates, Inc.)	150
Chemname™ (DIALOG Information Services, Inc. and Chemical Abstracts Service)	138
Chemsearch™ (DIALOG Information Services, Inc. and Chemical Abstracts Service)	138
Chemsis™ (DIALOG Information Services, Inc. and Chemical Abstracts Service)	138
Chemzero™ (DIALOG Information Services, Inc. and Chemical Abstracts Service)	138
Claims™ Compound Registry (IFI/Plenum Data Co.)	95
Paperchem (Institute of Paper Chemistry)	65
Scisearch® (Institute for Scientific Information)	165
TSCA Initial Inventory (DIALOG Information Services, Inc. and Environmental Protection Agency, Office of Toxic Substances)	45
Agriculture and Nutrition	
Agricola (National Agricultural Library)	35
BIOSIS Previews (BioSciences Information Service)	65
CAB Abstracts (The Commonwealth Agricultural Bureaux)	55
CRIS/USDA (U.S. Dept. of Agriculture)	35
Foods Science and Technology Abstracts (International Food Information Service)	65
Foods Adlibra (Komp Information Services)	55
Medicine and Biosciences	
BIOSIS Previews (BioSciences Information Service)	65
CA SEARCH (Chemical Abstracts Service)	68

Table 6.3 Online Databases Offered by DIALOG Information Services, Inc.[1] and Their Online Connect Time Rates, July 1983 (cont.)

Database (Supplier)	Online Connect Time Rate (per hour)
Chemical Exposure (Chemical Effects Information Center, Oak Ridge National Laboratory)	45
Chemname™ (DIALOG Information Services, Inc. and Chemical Abstracts Service)	138
Chemsearch™ (DIALOG Information Services, Inc. and Chemical Abstracts Service)	138
Chemsis™ (DIALOG Information Services, Inc. and Chemical Abstracts Service)	138
Chemzero™ (DIALOG Information Services, Inc. and Chemical Abstracts Service)	138
Excerpta Medica (Excerpta Medica)	75
Health Planning and Administration (U.S. National Library of Medicine)	35
International Pharmaceutical Abstracts (American Society of Hospital Pharmacists)	55
Life Sciences Collection (Cambridge Scientific Abstracts)	45
Medline (U.S. National Library of Medicine)	35
Mental Health Abstracts (IFI/Plenum Data Co.)[2]	55
Pharmaceutical News Index (Data Courier, Inc.)	95
Scisearch® (Institute for Scientific Information)	165
Telegen (Environment Information Center, Inc.)	90
Zoological Record (BioSciences Information Service and Zoological Society of London)	78
Energy and Environment	
Aptic (Manpower and Technical Information Branch, U.S. Environmental Protection Agency)	35
Aquaculture (National Oceanic and Atmospheric Administration)	35
Aqualine (Water Research Centre)	35
Aquatic Sciences and Fisheries Abstracts (NOAA/Cambridge Scientific Abstracts)	75
BIOSIS Previews (BioSciences Information Service)	65
CA Search (Chemical Abstracts Service)	68
DOE Energy (U.S. Dept. of Energy)	40
Electric Power Database (Electric Power Research Institute)	55

Table 6.3 Online Databases Offered by DIALOG Information Services, Inc.[1] and Their Online Connect Time Rates, July 1983 (cont.)

Database (Supplier)	Online Connect Time Rate (per hour)
Energyline® (Environment Information Center, Inc.)	90
Energynet® (Environment Information Center, Inc.)	90
Enviroline® (Environment Information Center, Inc.)	90
Environmental Bibliography (Environmental Studies Institute)	60
Oceanic Abstracts (Cambridge Scientific Abstracts)	73
Pollution Abstracts (Cambridge Scientific Abstracts)	73
Water Resources Abstracts (U.S. Dept. of the Interior)	45
Water Net (American Water Works Association)	80
Science and Technology	
BHRA Fluid Engineering (BHRA Fluid Engineering)	65
Compendex (Engineering Information, Inc.)	98
Ei Engineering Meetings (Engineering Information, Inc.	98
Geoarchive (Geosystems)	70
Georet (American Geological Institute)	82
INSPEC (The Institution of Electrical Engineers)	85
International Software Database (Imprint Software Ltd.)	60
ISMEC (Cambridge Scientific Abstracts)	73
Mathfile (American Mathematical Society)	55
Meteorological and Geoastrophysical Abstracts (American Meteorological Society)	95
Microcomputer Index™ (Microcomputer Information Services)	45
NTIS (National Technical Information Service, U.S. Dept. of Commerce)	45
Scisearch (Institute for Scientific Information)	165
SPIN (American Institute of Physics)	35
SSIE Current Research (National Technical Information Service, U.S. Dept of Commerce)	78
Standards and Specifications (National Standards Association, Inc.)	65
TRIS (U.S. Dept. of Transportation and Transportation Research Board)	40
Weldasearch (The Welding Institute)	75

Table 6.3 Online Databases Offered by DIALOG Information Services, Inc.[1] and Their Online Connect Time Rates, July 1983 (cont.)

Database (Supplier)	Online Connect Time Rate (per hour)
Materials Sciences	
CA Search (Chemical Abstracts Service)	68
Chemname (DIALOG Information Services, Inc. and Chemical Abstracts Service)	138
Chemsearch (DIALOG Information Services, Inc. and Chemical Abstracts Service)	138
Chemsis (DIALOG Information Services, Inc. and Chemical Abstracts Service)	138
Chemzero (DIALOG Information Services, Inc. and Chemical Abstracts Service)	138
METADEX (American Society for Metals)	80
Nonferrous Metals Abstracts (British Nonferrous Metals Technology Centre)	45
Paperchem (Institute of Paper Chemistry)	65
Surface Coatings Abstracts (Paint Research Association of Great Britain)	65
Textile Technology Digest (Institute of Textile Technology)	65
World Aluminum Abstracts (American Society for Metals)	50
World Textiles (Shirley Institute)	55
Patents and Trademarks	
CA Search (Chemical Abstracts Service)	68
CLAIMS™/Citation (Search Check, Inc. and IFI/Plenum Data Co.)	95
CLAIMS™/Class (IFI/Plenum Data Co.)	95
CLAIMS Compound Registry (IFI/Plenum Data Co.)	95
CLAIMS™/U.S. Patent Abstracts 1950-1970 (IFI/Plenum Data Co.)	95
CLAIMS™/U.S. Patent Abstracts 1971-1981 (IFI/Plenum Data Co.)	95
CLAIMS™/U.S. Patent Abstracts 1982-present (IFI/Plenum Data Co.)	95
CLAIMS™/U.S. Patent Abstracts Weekly (IFI/Plenum Data Co.)	95
CLAIMS™/UNITERM (IFI/Plenum Data Co.)	300

Table 6.3 Online Databases Offered by DIALOG Information Services, Inc.[1] and Their Online Connect Time Rates, July 1983 (cont.)

Database (Supplier)	Online Connect Time Rate (per hour)
Patlaw (Bureau of National Affairs, Inc.)	120
Trademarkscan™ (Thomson and Thomson)[3]	[3] |//
Business/Economics	
Bibliographic	
ABI/Inform (Data Courier, Inc.)	73
Adtrack (Corporate Intelligence Inc.)	95
Arthur D. Little/Online (Arthur D. Little Decision Resources)	90
Chemical Industry Notes (American Chemical Society)	74
Economic Literature Index (American Economic Association)	75
Economics Abstracts International (Learned Information, Ltd.)	65
FIND/SVP Reports and Studies Index (FIND/SVP)	65
HARFAX Industry Data Sources (Harfax Database Publishing)	75
Harvard Business Review (John Wiley & Sons, Inc.)[3]	[3]
Insurance Abstracts (University Microfilms International)	55
Management Contents® (Management Contents, Inc.)	80
Pharmaceutical News Index (Data Courier, Inc.)	95
PTS Annual Reports Abstracts (Predicasts, Inc.)	120
PTS F&S Indexes (Predicasts, Inc.)	95
PTS PROMT (Predicasts, Inc.)	95
Standard & Poor's News (Standard & Poor's Corp.)	85
Standard & Poor's News Daily (Standard & Poor's Corp.)	85
Trade and Industry Index™ (Information Access Co.)	85
Numeric	
BI/DATA Forecasts (Business International Corp.)	85
BI/DATA Time Series (Business International Corp.)	85
BLS Consumer Price Index (Bureau of Labor Statistics, U.S. Dept. of Labor)	45

Table 6.3 Online Databases Offered by DIALOG Information Services, Inc.[1] and Their Online Connect Time Rates, July 1983 (cont.)

Database (Supplier)	Online Connect Time Rate (per hour)
BLS Employment, Hours, and Earnings (Bureau of Labor Statistics, U.S. Dept. of Labor)	45
BLS Labor Force (Bureau of Labor Statistics, U.S. Dept. of Labor)	45
BLS Producer Price Index (Bureau of Labor Statistics, U.S. Dept. of Labor)	45
Disclosure II (Disclosure Inc.)	60
PTS International Forecasts (Predicasts, Inc.)	95
PTS International Time Series (Predicasts, Inc.)	95
PTS U.S. Forecasts (Predicasts, Inc.)	95
PTS U.S. Time Series (Predicasts, Inc.)	95
U.S. Exports (U.S. Dept. of Commerce)	45
Directories	
Commerce Business Daily (Commerce Business Daily, U.S. Dept. of Commerce)	54
Disclosure II (Disclosure Inc.)	60
D&B-Dun's Market Identifiers 10+® (Dun's Marketing Services)	100
D&B-Million Dollar Directory (Dun's Marketing Services)	100
D&B-Principal International Businesses® (International Marketing Services, Dun & Bradstreet International)	100
EIS Industrial Plants (Economic Information Systems, Inc.)	90
EIS Nonmanufacturing Establishments (Economic Information Systems, Inc.	90
Electronic Yellow Pages-Construction Directory (Market Data Retrieval, Inc.)	60
Electronic Yellow Pages-Financial Services Directory (Market Data Retrieval, Inc.)	60
Electronic Yellow Pages-Manufacturers Directory (Market Data Retrieval, Inc.)	60
Electronic Yellow Pages-Professionals Directory (Market Data Retrieval, Inc.)	60
Electronic Yellow Pages-Retailers Directory (Market Data Retrieval, Inc.)	60

Table 6.3 Online Databases Offered by DIALOG Information Services, Inc.[1] and Their Online Connect Time Rates, July 1983 (cont.)

Database (Supplier)	Online Connect Time Rate (per hour)
Electronic Yellow Pages-Services Directory (Market Data Retrieval, Inc.)	60
Electronic Yellow Pages-Wholesalers Directory (Market Data Retrieval, Inc.)	60
Foreign Traders Index (U.S. Dept. of Commerce)	45
Trade Opportunities (U.S. Dept. of Commerce)	45
Trade Opportunities Weekly (U.S. Dept of Commerce)	45
Industry Specific	
Chemical Industry Notes (American Chemical Society)	74
Coffeeline (International Coffee Organization)	65
Foods Adlibra (Komp Information Services)	55
Insurance Abstracts (University Microfilms International)	55
Pharmaceutical News Index (Data Courier, Inc.)	95
Law and Government	
ASI (Congressional Information Service, Inc.)	90
CIS (Congressional Information Service, Inc.)	90
Chemical Regulations and Guidelines System (U.S. Interagency Regulatory Liason Group, CRC Systems, Inc.)	70
Chemlaw (Bureau of National Affairs, Inc. and Fein-Marquart Associates, Inc.)	150
Commerce Business Daily (Commerce Business Daily, U.S. Dept. of Commerce)	54
Congressional Record Abstracts (Capitol Services International)	75
Criminal Justice Periodicals Index (University Microfilms International)	55
Federal Index (Capitol Services International)	90
Federal Register Abstracts (Capitol Services International)	75
GPO Monthly Catalog (U.S. Government Printing Office)	35
GPO Publications Reference File (U.S. Government Printing Office)	35

Database Publishing: Print and Online   145

Table 6.3 Online Databases Offered by DIALOG Information Services, Inc.[1] and Their Online Connect Time Rates, July 1983 (cont.)

Database (Supplier)	Online Connect Time Rate (per hour)
Laborlaw (Bureau of National Affairs, Inc.)	120
Legal Resource Index (Information Access Co.)	90
NCJRS (National Criminal Justice Reference Service)	35
NTIS (National Technical Information Service, U.S. Dept. of Commerce)	45
Patlaw (Bureau of National Affairs, Inc.)	120
TSCA Initial Inventory (DIALOG Information Services, Inc. and Environmental Protection Agency, Office of Toxic Substances)	45
Current Affairs	
Chronolog Newsletter (DIALOG Information Retrieval Service)	15
Magazine Index™ (Information Access Co.)	80
National Newspaper Index™ (Information Access Co.)	80
Newsearch™ (Information Access Co.)	95
Online Chronicle (Online, Inc.)	35
PAIS International (PAIS, Inc.)	60
Standard and Poor's News (Standard & Poor's Corp.)	85
Standard and Poor's News Daily (Standard & Poor's Corp.)	85
UPI News (United Press International, Inc.)	85
World Affairs Report (California Institute of International Affairs)	90
Directories	
American Men and Women of Science (R.R. Bowker)	95
Biography Master Index (Gale Research Co.)	55
Career Placement Registry/Experienced Personnel (Career Placement Registry, Inc.)	50
Career Placement Registry/Student (Career Placement Registry, Inc.)	50
Encyclopedia of Associations (Gale Research Co.)	45
Marquis Who's Who (Marquis Who's Who, Inc.)	[4]
Ulrich's International Periodicals Directory (R.R. Bowker)	65

Table 6.3 Online Databases Offered by DIALOG Information Services, Inc.[1] and Their Online Connect Time Rates, July 1983 (cont.)

Database (Supplier)	Online Connect Time Rate (per hour)
Social Sciences and Humanities	
America: History and Life (ABC-Clio, Inc.)	65
Artbibliographies Modern (ABC-Clio, Inc.)	60
Child Abuse and Neglect (National Center on Child Abuse and Neglect, Children's Bureau, U.S. Dept. of Health and Human Services)	35
Family Resources Database (National Council on Family Relations and Inventory of Marriage and Family Literature Project)	[4]
Historical Abstracts (ABC-Clio, Inc.)	65
Information Science Abstracts (IFI/Plenum Data Co.)	[4]
Language and Language Behavior Abstracts (Sociological Abstracts, Inc.)	55
LISA (Learned Information Ltd.)	75
MLA Bibliography (Modern Language Association)	55
PAIS International (PAIS, Inc.)	60
Philosopher's Index (Philosophy Documentation Center)	55
Population Bibliography (University of North Carolina, Carolina Population Center)	55
Psycinfo (American Psychological Association)	55
Religion Index (American Theological Library Association)	[4]
RILM Abstracts (City University of New York, International RILM Center)	65
Social Scisearch® (Institute for Scientific Information)	110
Sociological Abstracts (Sociological Abstracts, Inc.)	55
United States Political Science Abstracts (University of Pittsburgh, NASA Industrial Applications Center)	65
World Affairs Report (California Institute of International Affairs)	90
Multidisciplinary	
Comprehensive Dissertation Index (University Microfilms International)	70
Conference Papers Index (Cambridge Scientific Abstracts)	73

Table 6.3 Online Databases Offered by DIALOG Information Services, Inc.[1] and Their Online Connect Time Rates, July 1983 (cont.)

Database (Supplier)	Online Connect Time Rate (per hour)
DIALINDEX™ (DIALOG Information Services, Inc.)	35
NTIS (National Technical Information Service, U.S. Dept. of Commerce)	45
Education	
AIM/ARM (The Center for Vocational Education. The Ohio State University)	25
ERIC (National Institute of Education and ERIC Processing and Reference Facility)	25
Exceptional Child Education Resources (The Council for Exceptional Children)	35
IRIS (U.S. Environmental Protection Agency Information Project, Ohio State University)	35
NICEM (National Information Center for Educational Media, U. of Southern California)	70
NICSEM/NIMIS (National Information Center for Special Education Materials)	35
U.S. Public School Directory (National Center for Educational Statistics)	35
Bibliography-Books and Monographs	
Book Review Index (Gale Research Co.)	55
Books in Print (R.R. Bowker)	65
DIALOG Publications (DIALOG Information Services, Inc.)	15
GPO Monthly Catalog (U.S. Government Printing Office)	35
GPO Publications Reference File (U.S. Government Printing Office)	35
LC MARC (U.S. Library of Congress)	45
REMARC (Carrollton Press)	85
Foundations and Grants	
Foundation Directory (The Foundation Center)	60
Foundation Grants Index (The Foundation Center)	60
Grants (Oryx Press)	60
National Foundations (The Foundation Center)	60

Table 6.3 Online Databases Offered by DIALOG Information Services, Inc.[1] and Their Online Connect Time Rates, July 1983 (cont.)

Database (Supplier)	Online Connect Time Rate (per hour)
Online Training and Practice	
ONTAP® ABI/INFORM (Data Courier, Inc. and DIALOG Information Services, Inc.)	15
ONTAP® CA SEARCH (Chemical Abstracts Service and DIALOG Information Services, Inc.)	15
ONTAP® Chemname (Chemical Abstracts Service and DIALOG Information Services, Inc.)	15
ONTAP® COMPENDEX (Engineering Information, Inc. and DIALOG Information Services, Inc.)	15
ONTAP® DIALINDEX (DIALOG Information Services, Inc.)	15
ONTAP® ERIC (ERIC and DIALOG Information Services, Inc.)	15
ONTAP® INSPEC (The Institution of Electrical Engineers and DIALOG Information Services, Inc.)	15
ONTAP® Magazine Index (Information Access Co. and DIALOG Information Services, Inc.)	15
ONTAP® MEDLINE (U.S. National Library of Medicine and DIALOG Information Services, Inc.)	15
ONTAP® PTS PROMT (Predicasts, Inc. and DIALOG Information Services, Inc.)	15

[1]DIALOG Information Services, Inc. is a subsidiary of Lockheed Corp.
[2]Through 1982 database was supplied by National Clearinghouse for Mental Health Information, National Institute of Mental Health.
[3]Forthcoming database.
[4]Price to be announced.
Source: DIALOG Information Services, Inc., July 1983.

Among the company's other print products are *Energy Abstracts* and *Bioengineering Abstracts*, monthly collections of abstracts related to energy engineering and bioengineering. Generally, these abstracts also appear in *Engineering Index Monthly*.

COMPENDEX, COMPuterized ENgineering inDEX, is a machine-readable form of the *Ei Monthly* and *Annual*. It contains over 1 million abstracts—61% are journal articles; 30%, conference proceedings; and 9% reports and monographs—arranged and cross-referenced under more than 12,000 indexing terms. All data from 1969 to the present are online, and the database is growing by about 10,000 abstracts each month.

In 1982 Ei launched Ei Engineering Meetings (EIMET), a database providing an index to the published proceedings of approximately 2000 domestic and international engineering and technical conferences, symposia, meetings and colloquia held each year. The database contains about 150,000 records; in 1984 about 100,000 records will be added.

Vendors pay Ei $10,500 each annually for the right to sell material from COMPENDEX or EIMET plus a royalty of $50 per connect hour. Corporations pay $8000 annually for the right to reproduce the information internally and use it for any purpose they wish; however, they cannot sell it. In this manner Ei distinguishes between an information vendor and a customer that wishes to use its data internally.

In 1980, Ei established the Engineering Information Search Service (EISS), an information retailing service created to service engineering companies, consultants and colleges that lack trained information researchers. EISS will locate information on nearly any subject, whether it be the cost-of-living index in Pakistan or the avoidance of fatigue failure in offshore steel structures. It will obtain printed copies of any articles requested by the customer and will even translate articles available only in the author's native language. The service charges a base fee of $75 for each customer inquiry, but can be considerably higher, depending on charges for long distance telephone calls and computer connect time.

In 1980, Ei's revenues totaled $3.3 million; $2.4 million, or nearly 75%, was derived from print publications and the remaining $875,000 came from online services.

Institute for Scientific Information

The Institute for Scientific Information (ISI) is the only commercial publisher of sci-tech bibliographic information that deals with journal literature. It publishes several print services of which *Current Contents, Science Citation Index* (SCI) and *Social Sciences Citation Index* (SSCI) are among the best known.

Current Contents is a weekly pocket-sized publication containing tables of contents from about 1000 of the world's leading journals and from over 700 multi-authored books. Each issue is published in seven editions, including Clinical Practice; Engineering, Technology and Applied Sciences; and Physical, Chemical and Earth Sciences. Each edition is priced at $245 per year.

Science Citation Index, issued six times a year, is the world's only citation index to the complete range of sci-tech literature. Citation indexing, pioneered by ISI, identifies and groups together all newly published items that have referenced the same earlier work. Thus, the earlier document becomes, in effect, an indexing term useful in retrieving current papers on the same subject. It is also a means of identifying influential authors and articles by seeing how frequently they are cited in subsequent literature. In addition to the citation index, SCI includes three other indexes. Over 560,000 records are added annually, including every item in over 3300 scientific and technical journals. The annual cost for this index is $5200.

Social Sciences Citation Index, issued three times a year, provides the same type of indexing services for social sciences literature at a cost of $2300 per year. SSCI indexes more than 129,000 items from over 1400 leading social science journals. In addition, articles from more than 3200 scientific and technical journals are selected for their relevance to the social sciences.

ISI also publishes several other indexes as well as a number of services in the chemical field; it operates several current awareness services and a document retrieval service for articles reported, abstracted or indexed by ISI services.

Until November 1981, ISI operated only two online services: Scisearch and Social Scisearch. These services are essentially the online versions of the two major hard-copy indexes. Scisearch is available from Lockheed, while Social Scisearch can be accessed through Lockheed and BRS. In November 1981, ISI introduced three new online products: ISI/BIOMED™, ISI/ISTP&B™ (Index to Scientific & Technical Proceedings & Books) and ISI/CompuMath™.

The ISI/BIOMED database is drawn from the SCI database and includes all significant articles, meeting abstracts, letters, editorials, review papers, etc. dating back to 1979 from over 1400 biomedical journals. ISI/ISTP&B is the only multidisciplinary online database to the proceedings and monographs in nearly every scientific and technical discipline. The service annually covers about 3500 proceedings and 1650 multi-authored books, for a total of 142,000 records.

ISI/CompuMath covers the literature of mathematics, computer science, statistics, operations research and related disciplines, such as mathematical physics and econometrics. It includes the ISI/CompuMath online database and the *CompuMath Citation Index*. The database covers 1976 to the present and indexes every item from over 380 key journals in mathematics, computer science and related disciplines. It also covers relevant articles selected from over 6500 other journals in the sciences, social sciences and arts and humanities. The *CompuMath Citation Index*, published three times a year, covers the material found on the database.

Since 1981 ISI has introduced ISI/GeoSciTech, which covers the literature of geosciences/geotechnology, petroleum science, oceanography/marine technology, metallurgy/mining, mineralogy, meteorology/atmospheric science and related disciplines. The database covers 1978 to the present, indexing every significant item from 400 key geosciences journals plus relevant articles selected from an additional 6300 journals in the sciences, social sciences and arts and humanities.

Until February 29, 1984 these databases were available from the ISI Search Network. At present they are available through DIMDI, a West German vendor. With the exception of research front information, ISI/BIOMED and ISI/CompuMath data are also available through Scisearch or Social Scisearch. They are no longer available through the ISI Search Network.

In 1980, ISI's sales reached $20 million, of which $10 million was derived from its two major indexes and their online counterparts; online services probably accounted for $1 million of the total. About $10 million, or 50% of company sales, were to customers abroad.

National Library of Medicine

The National Library of Medicine (NLM), a part of the National Institute of Health, in turn a division of the U.S. Dept. of Health and Human Services, is the world's largest research library in a single scientific and professional field.

NLM's principal hard-copy publication, *Index Medicus*, has been published since 1879. It is a monthly index of references to journal articles from 2500 worldwide medical journals and runs approximately 1400 pages and 25,000 references each month. NLM also publishes *Abridged Index Medicus*, a monthly index covering about 100 English-language journals and designed for individual practitioners and small hospital and clinic libraries, as well as several other print publications.

MEDLARS (Medical Literature Analysis and Retrieval System) was established by NLM in 1964 for rapid bibliographic access to its biomedical data and was one of the first major machine-readable databases to be made available online nationwide. MEDLARS is the name given to NLM's entire computerized literature retrieval system and consists of 20 databases, including MEDLINE, TOXLINE, POPLINE and CHEMLINE.

MEDLINE, begun in late 1971, is the largest and most important database on the MEDLARS system. It is essentially an online version of *Index Medicus*; however, it contains articles from an additional 500 journals. Moreover, although *Index Medicus* only contains title, author and source data, MEDLINE also includes English-language abstracts if they appeared in the journal and if the publisher gives permission for their inclusion; thus, over 40% of the references in MEDLINE include abstracts. While the entire MEDLARS database contains over 6 million references, MEDLINE usually consists of an average of 800,000 references that cover the latest two to three years of data; over 250,000 records are added to MEDLINE each year.

MEDLARS is available through a nationwide network of NLM centers located at about 3500 universities, medical schools, hospitals, government agencies and commercial organizations. As of October 1, 1983, usage fees are charged on an algorithm that takes into account the amount of connect time, the number of characters sent to the terminal and the number of computer work units used, rather than a straight connect-hour fee. Generally, the fees average about $22 per hour in prime time (9 a.m. to 5 p.m.) and $15 in non-prime time.

Vendors pay NLM an annual lease fee of $20,000 plus $4 per hour for each hour of usage recorded. Sixty percent of MEDLINE use is directly through MEDLARS, however. In fiscal 1982, there were 2.3 million searches of the MEDLARS database, and in fiscal 1983 this figure exceeded 2.4 million. MEDLINE, with 784,625 searches, accounted for 34.8% of all MEDLARS searches in 1982. Billings for the entire MEDLARS system totaled $3.8 million in fiscal 1982.

Chemical Abstracts Service

Chemical Abstracts Service (CAS), formed in 1907 by the American Chemical Society, is today the society's largest staff division; it abstracts and indexes close to 500,000 papers, patents, books and other documents every year. CAS claims to be the only comprehensive abstracting and indexing service in chemistry outside the U.S.S.R. To create its database, CAS monitors some 12,000 sci-tech periodicals from over 150 countries in more than 50 languages, patent documents issued by 26 nations and two international bodies, plus conference proceedings, dissertations, government reports and books from all over the world.

In order to be selected for abstracting and indexing by CAS, a paper or patent must contain new information that is relevant to chemistry or chemical engineering. About 250 of the 12,000 periodicals monitored are abstracted and indexed in their entirety; papers are selected from 8500 different publications in any one year and from close to 12,000 periodicals over a five-year period. In 1982, CAS added 457,789 abstracts to its database to achieve a total of 9.5 million abstracts.

The most comprehensive and best known of CAS' publications is *Chemical Abstracts* (CA) which, it claims, is universally recognized as the "key to the world's chemical literature." It is the largest abstracting journal serving a single scientific discipline. Some 8000 to 9000 abstracts are published each week in issues that are about one-half the size of the Manhattan telephone directory. The abstracts are organized into 80 subject sections, which fall into five broad groupings: biochemistry; organic chemistry; macromolecular chemistry; applied chemistry and chemical engineering; and physical, inorganic and analytical chemistry. Each issue is indexed by author, patent number and key words. A one-year subscription to CA, including the weekly issues and *Volume Indexes*, costs $7500.

At five-year intervals the *Volume Indexes* are merged and republished as a *Collective Index* to the period's chemical and chemical engineering literature. CA's 11th *Collective Index* (1982-1986), which will begin publication in 1987, will consist of about 86 volumes and will provide access to an estimated 2.8 million documents; it will contain about 146,000 pages. Prepublication prices range from $12,600 to $16,200, depending on year of purchase. Price upon publication is expected to be $18,000.

CAS also publishes *Chemical Industry Notes* (CIN), a weekly compilation of abstracts from over 80 key trade and business periodicals published in nine countries. This publication is intended for chemists, chemical engineers and others engaged in management, production or marketing; it is priced at $1000. In addition, CAS publishes many other hard-copy services and reference works, including *CAS Source Index* (CASSI), a compilation of bibliographic and library holdings data for about 50,000 publications.

In 1981, CAS and BioSciences Information Service began joint publication of BIOSIS/CAS Selects. This series of 31 biweekly publications contains abstracts from biological and chemical literature, such as the biochemistry of fermented foods, interferon or schizophrenia.

Many of the print services published by CAS are also available in machine-readable format, and several are online, including CIN and CA SEARCH, the online version of CA. Although CIN online contains the actual abstracts carried by the hard-copy service, CA SEARCH carries only the bibliographic and index data on the 6 million documents abstracted in CA since 1967.

In 1980, CAS began producing CAS ONLINE, a service which enables users to perform online searches of chemical substance information in the CAS Registry System, a computer file of over 6 million substances and over 9 million names referenced in CA since 1965. Through CAS ONLINE a searcher can identify substances that share certain structural characteristics. Answers are displayed as two-dimensional structure diagrams, each accompanied by a molecular formula, CAS Registry number and other data, on the screen of a compatible graphics terminal. In late 1983 CAS ONLINE became a "subject" search system as well. The expanded system may be accessed by subject index terms, keywords, bibliographic data and Registry Numbers in addition to structure searching. Answers can include CA abstracts and/or index entries.

CAS ONLINE is the first computer file offered by CAS that can be directly searched by individuals. Because CAS ONLINE is based on a large, complex nonbibliographic database, the technology required to make that database available in an efficient, effective manner is different from the technology currently used for bibliographic files. Since it builds and maintains the chemical substance database used in CAS ONLINE, CAS concluded it was best qualified to provide useful access to this file and that adequate service could not be provided through the licensing of the CAS chemical substance files.

In addition to the on-line services offered by CAS, its parent, the American Chemical Society, began offering the full text of 18 journals through BRS in June 1983. The initial file contained over 29,000 articles dating back to 1980.

In 1980, CAS revenue totaled an estimated $42 million, of which $32 million was derived from print services, $4 million from machine-readable products and $6 million from government contracts and other sources.

Excerpta Medica

Excerpta Medica (EM), part of the Associated Scientific Publishers group of companies within Elsevier, a Netherlands publishing house, is (together with NLM) one of the two most important publishers of medical databases in the world, and therefore deserves mention in this book. Excerpta Medica was begun by a group of physicians during 1946 and 1947 as an independent Dutch foundation; in the early 1970s, it became part of the Elsevier family of companies. It publishes abstract bulletins, drug literature bibliographies and core journals as products of a computerized database of information from biomedical journals. All editorial work, with the exception of some of the abstracting and translating and a certain amount of linguistic supervision, takes place in Amsterdam. EM's database currently includes about 2 million bibliographic references. It regularly screens over 3500 biomedical journals; over 10,000 pages are screened daily. The screening process results in about 250,000 citations and 150,000 abstracts annually.

The database is divided into 43 subject areas, each of which is reflected in a printed abstract journal. Each of the 43 abstract journals is concerned with a particular specialty across the range of human medicine and includes such nonmedical topics as health economics and hospital management. Besides the abstract journals, which are issued 10 to 30 times per year, EM also publishes two drug-related literature indexes.

In addition, EM publishes a series of nine core journals in fields such as pediatrics, clinical neurology an ophthalmology. These publications provide physicians with an overview of the most important published clinical research in their fields within one month of publication.

In August 1978 the EM database went online through Dialog, covering all data from mid-1974 to the present. The file corresponds to the printed abstract journals and literature indexes of EM plus an additional 100,000 records annually that do not appear in the hard-copy publications. The online database is updated monthly, with about 20,000 new abstracts and citations. The database is also carried by BRS and two other vendors.

EM also puts abstracts from nearly 300 medical journals, including *New England Journal of Medicine* and *Journal of the American Medical Association* into a clinical literature database for the AMA's AMA/NET medical information network. The service, called EMPIRES, is connected with GTE Telenet's MINET medical information network. The database dates back to 1981; 50,000 new citations and abstracts are added each year.

In addition to its database activities, EM plans, develops and manages medical seminars and symposia; organizes medical congresses and publishes proceedings; and publishes patient education aids and audio-visual materials.

BioSciences Information Service

BioSciences Information Service (BIOSIS), an independent nonprofit organization, is the world's largest English-language abstracting and indexing service for biological and biomedical research. The entire BIOSIS file presently contains over 5 million reports. Its annual coverage totals 335,000 items drawn from over 9000 serials, books, monographs, conference proceedings, etc.

The two major hard-copy publications produced by BIOSIS are *Biological Abstracts* (BA) and *Biological Abstracts/RRM* (BA/RRM). BA, issued semimonthly and published since 1927, provides bibliographic citations and English-language abstracts of basic research papers from primary biological and biomedical journals. About 185,000 abstracts are published per year (7700 per issue), at an annual cost of $2450. BA/RRM, which is issued semimonthly, includes letters, notes, symposia papers, meetings abstracts, trade journal items, etc. It is composed of full bibliographic citations plus descriptive words, concepts and taxonomic identifiers. BA/RRM contains about 6250 citations in every issue, and during 1983 is expected to provide citations for 150,000 items; a year's subscription is $1225.

BIOSIS also publishes three specialized monthly abstract journals, each containing 12,000 to 13,000 abstracts annually derived from the BIOSIS database—*Abstracts of Entomology*, *Abstracts of Mycology* and *Abstracts on Health Effects of Environmental Pollutants*. The services cost $130, $135 and $160, respectively. The organization also publishes *BioResearch Today*, a series of 14 monthly abstract journals selling for $75 per year and covering specific topics, such as birth defects, carcinogenesis, and food additives and residues, and, in 1981, began the joint publication of BIOSIS/ CAS Selects with Chemical Abstracts Service. This series of 31 biweekly publications contains abstracts from biological and chemical literature.

In 1980 BIOSIS agreed to publish *Zoological Record* (ZR) jointly with the Zoological Society of London. The Society continues to exercise editorial control and define the scope of the publication; however, BIOSIS has assumed responsibility for its management and production. ZR, the world's oldest indexing service, has been in existence since 1864. Published annually, it is the world's largest taxonomic index to zoological literature. In 1982 over 62,000 items from more than 6000 journals and other documents were placed in five indexes: author, subject, geographical, palaeontological and systematic. ZR may be purchased in its entirety or any of its 27 sections. The price for the entire volume is $1550.

In addition to several machine-readable services, BIOSIS offers BIOSIS Previews, BA Abstracts on Tape (BAT) and Zoological Record online. Previews is the online version of citations and index items from BA and BA/RRM; over 300,000 items are added each year. It is available online through Lockheed, SDC, BRS and eight other vendors throughout the world. BAT contains the full English-language text of the abstracts appearing in BA since July 1976. It is carried online by at least six systems. *Zoological Record* went online in 1982 and covers the zoological literature of 1978 and 1979. It is updated bimonthly.

DISTRIBUTION

Because of the differences in format, hard-copy and online services are marketed in different manners.

Hard-Copy Services

Print services are generally sold by direct mail, space advertising, and exhibits at educational seminars, conferences, conventions, etc. Some organizations, such as ISI and CAS, also employ salesmen, especially when selling expensive products such as ISI's *Science Citation Index.* CAS' sales force, which consists of five salespeople plus a sales manager, sells the full line of CAS services—print and online—and concentrates on the development of large commercial accounts.

The largest customers for print services are generally libraries and academic institutions. An established service usually finds that renewals constitute the majority of business; renewal rates are high—in some cases, over 90%. Over 2000 libraries worldwide are the primary customers for the major indexes published by ISI. However, in order to help smaller libraries provide an improved line of reference services to their patrons, ISI began a Library Grant Program in 1970 under which libraries can get discounts of up to 75% off list price.

Online Services

In most cases, online database services are offered to the user through a middleman or database vendor. The vendor makes potential customers aware of the advantages of online search and tries to convince them that it provides the best service and variety of databases. The producer, on the other hand, builds up the use of his own database via advertising, seminars, convention exhibits and other forms of merchandising directed toward the end user.

A trend may be originating, however, which will involve direct offering of online databases to customers by their producers, as witnessed by CAS' CAS ONLINE. In the past, database producers looked on vendors as the most efficient means of distribution. Now there is a feeling that the producer has more control with a private file; he can set all the terms and conditions for the user and at the same time can obtain necessary information about the use of the database, including identification of users. This feedback can be used to improve the existing product and create derivative products.

In addition, database producers have been receiving some 30% to 50% of the revenue from the use of their databases online, with the remainder going to the vendor. By offering the database directly, the producer receives the entire fee paid by the customer to use its file and does not have to share revenues with the vendor. It should be noted, however, that when a producer offers a database directly, he must also bear the costs of mounting and maintaining the file online, as well as of marketing the file.

International Sales

International sales are important to both the print and online sectors of the TSM database market. Many of the major producers of print databases find that a large part of their sales are to foreign customers; therefore, they employ sales representatives or agents in most parts of the world. Chemical Abstracts Service, for instance, has agreements with organizations in the United Kingdom, West Germany, France and Japan, under which these companies function as marketing representatives for CAS services.

Databases are also marketed abroad by online database vendors. BIOSIS Previews is offered by organizations located in Canada, Bulgaria, the Federal Republic of Germany, Italy, Switzerland, Australia and Japan. CA SEARCH is marketed by vendors in the United Kingdom, Canada, France, Italy, Japan and Switzerland, and is offered on magnetic tape by organizations located in 14 other countries, including Czechoslovakia, Israel, Korea and South Africa.

ECONOMICS OF DATABASE PUBLISHING

A comprehensive database service requires a large investment to start and maintain. For example, the CA database, which is characterized by its comprehensiveness, is said to cost well over $30 million annually to generate and operate. There is no homogeneity of costs in the database business because of variations in coverage. Among the factors affecting costs are the type of data involved, the cost of collection, the comprehensiveness of the data, the "value added" to the information and the methods by which the database is marketed and delivered.

Fixed costs for both online and hard-copy database publishing lie in acquiring, analyzing and recording information. Since, in the past, most producers of TSM databases compiled them for purposes other than online searches, their sale through a vendor represented a relatively small source of supplementary income. Many producers of TSM databases are not-for-profit organizations whose major business is the publication of print databases; commercial publishers also derive the major portion of their revenues from publishing the output of their databases in printed format. Thus, because the online service is often considered a derivative or by-product of an already existing hard-copy service, frequently it has not carried its proportionate share of costs; in effect, the print product has subsidized the online service. As online services have become more significant contributors to revenue, however, producers have been forced to allocate costs in a more formal manner.

Economics of a Hard-Copy Service

Industry experts differ in their opinions as to whether the major costs of a printed service are editorial or stem from production, printing and mailing. Some point out that editorial costs may be substantial because of the volume of indexing and abstracting that is involved in many services; however, often a large part of this work is performed by volunteers at no charge. Others stress that production, printing and mailing costs are also considerable, primarily because of the thousands of pages involved in the publications issued by many of the services.

When more than one service is published by the same firm, as is usually the case, publishing economies occur in paper, printing, photocomposition and staffing. Since the same database is normally used by several different services, the high costs of obtaining and processing the data can be spread over a larger base. Derivative services, however, which have a relatively small number of customers and are comparatively low-priced, may not be able to benefit from the economies of scale available to a large service. In addition, they may require more than their proportionate share of overhead.

Economics of Online Database Services

A computer-based information service needs a sizable investment of capital in order to create and maintain a database. However, in the TSM field, unlike the business information field, many online products are derivatives of hardcopy services that have been published for many years. Thus, as mentioned above, the initial costs of gathering, analyzing and processing the data were incurred by the print services and, in many cases today, are still considered part of the costs of the print service.

An online service is not subjected to the paper and printing costs incurred by a hard-copy service; if it is derived from a print product that uses computerized typesetting, the material is already in a form that can be delivered online. A service that is marketed by a vendor may have no fulfillment or distribution costs; however, a sizable marketing investment may be necessary. (As discussed above, while a producer promotes the use of his own database through advertising and merchandising directed toward the end user, the vendor must find ways to educate potential customers as to the advantages of online searching and try to convince them that the best service and greatest variety of databases are available through his particular company.)

160   TECHNICAL, SCIENTIFIC AND MEDICAL PUBLISHING

Royalties

Generally, when a vendor markets an online service, the producer of the service is entitled to royalties from its use. The producer charges the vendor a set fee, and the vendor, in turn, may charge whatever he wishes for the use of the service. For example, the American Psychological Association charges $15 per connect hour for PsycINFO; however, DIALOG offers it to the public for $55 per connect hour. Similarly, while CAS charges $30 per connect hour for CA SEARCH, DIALOG charges its customers $68 per connect hour. The National Library of Medicine, on the other hand, does not charge its vendors royalties for the use of the MEDLARS database; however, it is a government-sponsored service.

Price Sensitivity

Printed database services are apparently encountering significant price resistance, probably because their major customers tend to be libraries and these institutions are currently facing shrinking budget problems. Such customers have the option of switching to an online service and being charged according to usage.

Despite price increases, the use of online databases appears to be rising. Ei, for example, has raised its prices from $16 per connect hour in 1979 to $50 in 1984. Yet these increases do not appear to have interfered with its growth with respect to royalty income or online usage.

Pricing and the Migration from Print to Online

Database producers use the term "migration" to refer to customers dropping subscriptions to printed services in favor of online access. The problem is to know whether declining subscriptions are a result of increased online availability, or whether they would have declined in any event. Observers point out that most established hard-copy TSM products are mature services that do not grow substantially; they remain flat or lose a small amount of sales each year by attrition. New customers may be unable to afford a print service with all the necessary back issues; however, the corresponding online service will provide it with past as well as current data. Library budgets have also been decreasing, a factor that undoubtedly has a bearing on declining hard-copy sales; a study conducted by Ei indicated that from 1966 to 1980 subscribers to its print products declined 16%, or an average of about 1.1% per year, from 2500 in 1966 to 2100 in 1980. Finally, because of the form in which online usage information is received from the vendor, it is difficult to analyze the data in order to determine whether some sort of migration does exist.

On balance, it is probably likely that some degree of migration from print to online is occurring; however, it is a gradual movement rather than a plummeting drop. Those users that do migrate to online generally do so because of the high cost of the print service, but generally they find a way to obtain the printed information also, usually by sharing with local sources.

The producer of an online file has the problem of securing adequate compensation for his effort, especially if the development and maintenance of the underlying database have been supported by subscribers to the printed service. As these subscribers migrate to the online service, they reduce the revenue base that makes the service possible. Since the hard copy has up to this point subsidized the online database, the price of the online service must rise or resulting revenues will not be sufficient to pay the costs of producing the database.

Although the online rates for most bibliographic databases are currently based upon connect time use, this is not the ideal way to sell. A database should be priced to yield a profit to both the vendor and the producer regardless of the manner in which it is delivered.

The practice of charging by connect time use can result in lower publisher revenues, even if usage rises, as customers employ more advanced terminals and higher data transmission speeds. One solution is to shift toward user fees only partially based on connect time (in order to cover basic machine costs and discourage hogging of telecommunications lines) with a larger portion of the fee based on output; that is, the number of records retrieved.

As part of a program to link its charges more closely to the value of information rather than to the time it takes to transmit the content, in mid-1983 BRS announced a new 3¢ per print citation charge in addition to its standard hourly fees for all publicly available databases; in 1984 this charge was raised to 4¢. However, this method does not take into consideration a search that yields no hits but may still be extremely valuable to the searcher simply because it tells him that nothing has been published on a given subject.

In the early 1980s the Board of the American Chemical Society established several long-range financial objectives for CAS, including the generation of 4% net revenue above expenses over a five-year period and the reduction of the revenue contribution of the print version of *Chemical Abstracts* to no more than 50% of CAS income by 1984. This marketing orientation, which stipulated that revenue from non-print services must increase, placed all CAS products on a full-cost basis. CAS is said to have met its objectives.

In early 1984 CAS announced it would not license its file of computer-readable CA abstracts to other online vendors for several years because abstracts online might produce a more rapid loss of subscriptions to its printed services than have the other online CAS files. (CAS began offering online access to over 3.5 million chemical abstracts in January 1984 exclusively through CAS ONLINE, although bibliographic files and indexes dating back to 1967, known as CA SEARCH, are offered on other online retrieval services as well as through CAS ONLINE.) CAS said:

> "Subscriber migration from printed CA to online retrieval threatens the revenues needed to build the database from which we produce both printed CA and files for online services. In the past two years, print subscriptions to CA have declined at more than double the rate of the preceding decade. Our market research clearly indicates that a growing cause of the users deciding to discontinue their printed subscriptions is their increasing use of online retrieval. Royalties that we derive from the use of the CAS database by other vendors do not replace the revenues we lose from cancelled subscriptions to printed CA. In fact, we receive only about one-third of the money users pay online vendors for searching the CAS database."

The major database distributors such as Dialog, have long argued against raising hourly connect charges, claiming that this would cut into usage and harm everyone in the database field—publishers and vendors alike. Dialog has also claimed that there is no objective evidence to support the contention that online access hurts printed subscription sales. Nevertheless, connect charges are now rising steadily, and in some cases dramatically, as more publishers conclude that this is the only way to offset increased costs.

PROBLEMS IN TSM DATABASE PUBLISHING

Two major problems exist for companies involved in TSM database publishing: copyright violation and competition from the government. In addition, of course, rising costs are a problem, as they are throughout the TSM information industry.

Copyright Violations

Most copyright problems involving TSM databases center around two questions: Are online databases copyrightable? Are abstracts considered derivative works and, therefore, infringements of copyright in the absence of permissions from the owners of source material? There is also the fear that a user may, instead of taking a printout or display, capture data on a video cassette, video disc or minicomputer; he then has his own mini database he can use for repeated searches.

In an effort to deal with some of these problems, Chemical Abstracts Service now permits the "downloading" (capturing electronically) of data extracted from CAS online files and hard-copy services. With a downloading license, renewable annually, customers may capture up to 50,000 citations per year, including abstracts, index terms and other information associated with a cited document. For a single fee information captured in a given year may be stored and reused indefinitely within the customer's organization. External distribution or publishing of the information requires additional fees.

Similarly, BIOSIS permits the contents of *BIOSIS Previews* and *Zoological Record Online* databases to be downloaded for a one-time fee per record for the right to retain and use the data internally. Annual fees are based on type and number of records to be downloaded.

Legal experts differ as to what constitutes an infringement of databases. Many producers believe databases can be copyrighted, and feel that data printed out or displayed on a screen should carry a copyright symbol. Others believe protection lies with the contract rather than the copyright. A copyright gives strong initial protection for database products, but licensing agreements offer more control over the manner in which data are used. Lease or license arrangements typically specify that the producer retains ownership of the data, and the user agrees not to reproduce them.

In the past, publishers of primary information did not care if their data were abstracted or indexed, believing that this procedure gave the data additional exposure. Now, however, many publishers are aware of the revenues involved in online searching and are either putting up their database in full text or are indexing and abstracting it themselves. In addition, although at present many database producers obtain permission from the publisher to print an abstract, as full text begins to be carried online, these producers fear this permission may be construed to imply that royalty charges can be imposed. The revised Copyright Law does not cover the practice of abstracting; however, it is likely that primary publishers will begin to demand legislative relief from the practice of abstracting by anyone other than themselves.

Government Competition With the Private Sector

The federal government has from time to time preempted a market segment that private industry would prefer to serve, and past actions of the National Library of Medicine (NLM) are perhaps the best-known example.

In March 1975, NLM announced that it would provide all patrons direct access to MEDLINE and other database services. Until then, it had made its databases available to hospitals and research organizations directly while System Development Corp. (SDC) provided paid access for other users; the loss of MEDLINE revenues was estimated to have cost SDC more than $250,000 in annual billings. SDC sued the federal government, claiming that MEDLINE tapes were records and should be made available under the Freedom of Information Act; it alleged that the government had breached its contract by directly providing service to commercial customers. The court reviewing the case ruled, however, that since MEDLINE tapes are bibliographic, they are not considered records under the Freedom of Information Act, and further, that the contract was ambiguous. Although currently both BRS and Dialog are licensed to offer MEDLINE, NLM still has its own distribution network in competition with these private vendors.

Commercial publishers argue that government should undertake new services and create new products only if there is a complete absence of similar services in the private sector and that these products should be priced to recover full costs. For example, the American Psychological Association produces PsycINFO; yet the National Institute of Mental Health is generating a similar database containing some duplication. Whereas not-for-profit publishers may complain about government competition, the not-for-profits themselves are criticized by commercial publishers for receiving grants to create databases, which are then marketed in competition with privately funded services.

Although the Reagan Administration believes government should not get involved with projects the private sector is capable of undertaking, agencies like NLM have not changed long-standing ways of creating and disseminating information services. In addition, cutbacks in government research grants and in aid to higher education could well hurt commercial publishers as well as not-for-profits by reducing support for scholars and scientists who do research and then publish the results.

OUTLOOK FOR DATABASE PUBLISHING

It is likely that the market for online services in the TSM field will continue to grow at the expense of hard-copy publications. As the acceptance of its technology increases, online will become ever more important. Many managers or professionals who are over 40 are not accustomed to sitting down at a terminal to conduct a search. As they are replaced by younger personnel who have grown up with computers, this attitude will lessen. In addition, scientists and engineers use machine-readable bibliographic databases much more intensively than other professionals, business executives or the general public. Decreases in computer and telecommunications costs and the increasing availability of full-text databases are also favorable factors for the future.

Online databases are becoming economically more attractive to produce than printed versions. Print is dependent upon paper, ink, film, postage and other supplies affected by rising costs. As the price of hard-copy publications rises in response to these increased costs, their sales are bound to fall by comparison with their online counterparts. Eventually, however, in order to meet the costs of maintaining the database itself, prices of online databases will also be forced to rise.

Hard-copy services, especially those that are well managed, will continue to survive, although with little growth. There are many advantages to hard copy as opposed to online. It is difficult to thumb through an online product, and large files cannot be searched as readily online as in print. Online lacks the permanence and transportability of print, and it is difficult for an untrained searcher to use a terminal to retrieve information. Table 6.4 lists positive and negative factors affecting the future development of TSM databases.

Table 6.4 Factors Influencing Future Growth of Databases

Positive	Negative
1. Computer memory and telecommunications costs dropping.	1. Online prices do not reflect cost of database creation—must increase.
2. Only a fraction of scientists and engineers use services now—growth potential.	2. Library budgets declining in real terms.
3. Printing and postage costs rising rapidly for printed versions.	3. Markets for TSM information are mature.
4. New database distributors mean additional marketing push.	4. Online users must be trained.
5. International market can be developed.	5. Theft of data difficult to control.
6. Increasing number of full-text databases becoming available.	

Although the online market for TSM services will grow relative to hard copy, the absolute size of this market will increase rather slowly. The major databases are all up and online; the number of industry and nonprofit information centers which are primary markets for TSM information are limited; and the most likely customers have already been sold.

Database publishers may also add other data elements, such as numeric data, to their databases and may try to give the end users materials they do not currently receive online, such as material from the trade press, but if searching ever becomes so routine that every engineer has his own terminal, then growth will come from taking existing complex databases and making it simpler for the end users to search them. The greatest prospect for future growth lies in the development of new and unique services that will open up entire market opportunities.

7

Conclusions

The technical, scientific and medical (TSM) information industry underwent tremendous change during the 1970s and is still in the midst of transformation and growth. New information products are appearing constantly, and the computer has become increasingly important for the storage and delivery of information. At the same time, however, costs of all types have escalated; copyright violations have become a more pressing problem; and the traditional printed media have been affected by large increases in paper, printing and postage rates.

LEADING COMPANIES IN THE TSM INFORMATION MARKET

The market for TSM information is divided into five major areas: books, magazines and journals, newsletters, loose-leaf services and database publishing. Many of the larger companies, such as C.V. Mosby and Academic Press, are involved in both book and journal publishing, and a few companies are active in several sectors of the industry. The American Chemical Society, for example, publishes books, magazines, journals and databases, and Harper & Row is involved with books, journals and loose-leaf services. No one firm is dominant throughout the entire TSM industry, however.

Table 7.1 ranks the 10 leading TSM information companies by their 1980 revenues derived from TSM information services. In most cases estimates have been used because the companies themselves do not provide sufficiently detailed breakdowns. It can be seen that in 1980 the top five companies accounted for 14.1% of industry revenues, and the top 10 companies accounted for nearly one-fourth of industry sales. Thus, the industry is not highly concentrated, compared to such published segments as elementary-high school texts or mass market paperbacks. Profit margins before taxes for the publishing operations of these 10 companies, where available, ranged from 7.5% to 15.4%. It should be kept in mind, however, that in some cases these figures are for total publishing operations while in other cases, they are for professional publishing only.

Table 7.1 Estimated Revenues and Pretax Profit Margin of 10 Leading TSM Information Companies, 1980

Rank	Company	Revenue[1] (in millions)	Pretax Profit Margin[2]
1	The Times Mirror Co.[3]	$57	15.4%
2	McGraw-Hill, Inc.	54	13.9
2	Harcourt Brace Jovanovich/ Academic Press	54	8.7
3	American Chemical Society[4]	51	NA
4	CBS/W.B. Saunders & Co.	50	7.8
5	International Thomson Organisation Ltd.[5]	47	NA
6	John Wiley & Sons	43	12.1
7	Harper & Row, Publishers, Inc.	33	7.5
8	Springhouse Corp.[6]	25	NA
9	Waverly Press, Inc.[7]	23	11.1
	Total revenue, 10 companies	$438	
	Total industry revenue	$1879	
	Leading companies as percent of total industry	23.3%	

[1]Derived from technical, scientific and medical information services.
[2]Based on results for CBS/Publishing Group, McGraw-Hill's books and educational services group, Times Mirror's book publishing group, Harcourt's results for Academic Press and professional publishing, professional publishing results at Harper & Row, and publishing results at Waverly Press.
[3]The C.V. Mosby Co. and Year Book Medical Publishers.
[4]Includes Chemical Abstracts Service.
[5]Medical Economics Co. and Van Nostrand Reinhold.
[6]In 1983 Intermed Communications, Inc. changed its name to Springhouse Corp.
[7]The Williams & Wilkins Co.
NA: Not available.
Source: Company annual reports and Knowledge Industry Publications, Inc.

GROWTH OF TSM INFORMATION SERVICES

As the knowledge explosion continues in the TSM field, the need for the communication of this information increases accordingly. With every new discipline or twig of a major discipline, there comes a need for new books, journals, newsletters, databases, etc. to communicate the resulting data in an organized fashion.

Due to the increasing specialization taking place in the TSM field, information services are also becoming more specialized. Generally, the original services in a field cover a broad area, but as the field itself develops, narrow segments grow in importance, and new services arise that are devoted to these more specialized segments. It is also easier for a new service to gain a foothold in a market by catering to a narrow sector of a field rather than by competing head-to-head with a broad-based service. In most cases, the new service does not knock out the older established one, but instead the two tend to coexist and, in many instances, to expand the total market.

THE OUTLOOK FOR TSM INFORMATION SERVICES

During the 1984-1988 period, the TSM information field will probably witness the continued conversion of information services from print to electronic media. As online services become more affordable, and as more and more professionals become familiar with and, even more important, comfortable with their use, such services will become a more significant factor in the market. Increasing numbers of journals and other printed services will use photocomposition in their production or will publish simultaneously in a machine-readable format, such as magnetic tape, making the development of online services less expensive. The rising costs of paper and of postage may also lead to the development of additional electronic services rather than their print counterparts.

It is unlikely, however, that electronic media will make print services obsolete in the foreseeable future. When it comes to information that must be consulted and read, such as a lengthy article on a new medical treatment or the description of a new research technique, print on paper is the most flexible and convenient means of communication. Books, journals or newsletters are easily transportable and can be read anywhere; it would be impractical for a user to take a terminal with him wherever he went so that he could access an online service at any time. In addition, while everyone has access to print media, terminals are less accessible. Moreover, materials that are referred to frequently and contain a large volume of analytical content, such as loose-leaf medical services, are also unlikely candidates for computerization.

Computerized information retrieval will continue to make inroads, however, especially on extensive databases from which a user wishes to choose only isolated pieces of information at any one time. The computer will also be instrumental in the creation of more sophisticated database services than are delivered in print. Therefore, it will be easier to develop specialized reporting services for new sectors of the TSM field as well as indexing and abstracting services directed toward these areas.

There is great opportunity for expansion in the newsletter and loose-leaf service sectors of the TSM information market. Few newsletters serve the scientific and technical segments of this market, and it would also seem that a large potential market must exist for loose-leaf services on engineering and scientific subjects.

Individual companies in the TSM information business will, of course, continue to expand by raising prices, increasing sales or developing new products. To date, the opportunities for services in one sector of the TSM information industry to develop spin-offs using the same data in another sector of the industry have been largely untouched. However, as obtaining and processing data becomes ever more expensive, companies will begin to utilize these opportunities as a means of spreading costs over a larger base. Newsletters, for example, have a ready market of subscribers to whom they can sell research reports on subjects related to their newsletter coverage, while journals could publish books composed of past articles on a given field. Both newsletters and journals could place their entire issues on-line in full-text form.

International sales are an important factor in the market for nearly all TSM information products. English has become the world's second language and the common language of science and technology. Because U.S. technology is considered more advanced than that of other countries, TSM products from this country are generally widely accepted abroad. In recent years, however, foreign-owned firms, such as Pergamon Press, Elsevier North-Holland and Springer-Verlag, have established successful branches in this country. In 1981, British-owned International Thomson Organisation Ltd. established a U.S. operation in the TSM field with its acquisition of several companies in this sector, including Medical Economics Co. and Van Nostrand Reinhold. In addition, as countries such as Brazil and Japan become more advanced in their scientific research, they too will become a source of research results that may be published in the United States, but may also be published abroad and marketed in this country in competition with U.S.-published materials.

Growth by Industry Segment

Table 7.2 presents the estimated size of the market (by segment) for TSM

Table 7.2 Estimated and Projected Revenue of the Technical, Scientific and Medical Information Market, by Segment, 1982 and 1988

Segment	Estimated Revenue 1982 (In millions)	Segment as Percent of Total	Projected Revenue 1988 (In millions)	Segment as Percent of Total	Percent Increase 1982-1988
Magazines and journals (advertising and subscription revenue)	$893	38.7%	$1500	34.6%	68.0%
Database publishing	660	28.6	1570	36.3	137.9
Print	$535	23.2	850	19.6	58.9
Online	125	5.4	720	16.6	476.0
Technical, Scientific and Medical Books	700	30.3	1170	27.0	67.1
Newsletters	48	2.1	80	1.8	66.7
Loose-leaf services	6	0.3	10	0.2	66.7
Total market	$2307	100.0%	$4330	100.0%	87.7%

Note: Discrepancies in totals are due to rounding.
Source: Knowledge Industry Publications, Inc.

information services in 1982 and 1988. Projections for 1988 take into account the assumption that inflation will continue at an annual rate of 4% for the entire period.

Newsletters and loose-leaf services are expected to account for about the same portion of the market in 1988 as in 1982; however, magazines and journals, print database publishing and books will decline slightly in importance. Online database publishing will be the only sector to increase its market share, more than tripling in importance between 1982 and 1988. Online database publishing will also show the fastest rate of growth during this period.

In considering the outlook for growth of the TSM information market, it must be kept in mind that, because of the great importance of federal funds to research activities, any large change in funding by the federal government would have a significant effect on the amount of research conducted in the United States and, therefore, on the volume of information generated by this research.

8
Profiles of Major TSM Publishers

Academic Press
(Subsidiary of Harcourt Brace Jovanovich, Inc.)
111 Fifth Ave.
New York, NY 10003
(212) 741-6800

Imprints
Academic Press
Grune & Stratton

Representative Publications
Computers and Biomedical Research
Journal of Surgical Research
Virology

Academic Press, a subsidiary of Harcourt Brace Jovanovich, Inc. (HBJ), is part of the Academic Press and Professional Publishing segment of Harcourt Brace Jovanovich, Publishers, one of HBJ's three operating companies. Academic publishes treatises, monographs, series, textbooks, books and journals on technical, scientific and medical subjects, as well as books in the social sciences that have a scientific basis. The largest portion of its revenues is thought to be derived from titles in the fields of biological and medical science. Academic's subsidiary, Grune & Stratton, publishes books and journals on clinical medicine, psychology and special education.

Academic and Grune & Stratton publish a combined total of 731 titles in 1983. Academic aims for a broad international market and finds the European Economic Community countries and Japan to be its most important export markets.

Academic publishes 223 journals: 48 journals in the behavioral and social sciences; 66 journals in life sciences and biochemistry; 53 medical journals and 56 journals in mathematics and pure and applied sciences. The great majority of subscribers are libraries, with about half of the subscriptions going abroad.

In addition to Grune & Stratton, other subsidiaries of Academic Press include Johnson Reprint Corp., a publisher of facsimiles of out-of-print or rare sciences and humanities materials; and Grafacon, Inc., a phototypesetting plant primarily used for the company's journals.

TSM publishing accounts for two-thirds of Academic's estimated annual revenue of $75 million and is probably evenly divided between books and journals.

American Chemical Society
1155 Sixteenth St., N.W.
Washington, DC 20036
(202) 872-4600

Database Division:
Chemical Abstracts Service
2540 Olentangy River Rd.
P.O. Box 3012
Columbus, OH 43210
(614) 421-3600

Representative Publications and Services
Chemical & Engineering News
Analytical Chemistry
Journal of Chemical Information and Computer Sciences
Chemical Abstracts
Chemical Industry Notes
CA SEARCH
CAS ONLINE

The American Chemical Society (ACS), a not-for-profit organization, publishes books, monographs, magazines and journals in the chemistry field; its Chemical Abstracts Service (CAS) division publishes databases in both print and machine-readable formats. The smallest portion of revenue—$1.9 million, or 2.3%—generated by ACS' information services is derived from its book publishing operation, begun in 1949.

ACS prints a small number of monographs each year, as well as some 40 book titles, the majority of which are proceedings and symposia of the 128,000-member organization. Usually it prints about 1500 copies, and the book is not reprinted. Titles are sold by direct mail to members and others in the chemistry field, to libraries and to scientific and technical (sci-tech) bookstores. Sales to foreign countries account for 30% of sales.

The organization prints 19 periodicals—14 journals containing original research, two review journals, two publications with the characteristics of both magazines and journals and one magazine, *Chemical & Engineering*

News. The magazine, a weekly, is the society's official publication and is sent automatically to all members.

Prices for the 19 periodicals range from $13 to $60 for ACS members and $50 to $300 for nonmembers; in some instances there is also a nonmember (institutional) rate. *Analytical Chemistry*, with a circulation of 32,000 is ACS' largest journal in terms of both circulation size and advertising revenue. About 25% of combined journal and magazine revenue is derived from advertising; the remaining 75% comes from subscriptions, page charges, reprints and microfilm sales.

Twelve of the society's journals have voluntary page charges of $25 to $40; however, ACS hopes to phase them out in the future.

In 1983 ACS began offering the full text of 18 journals online through Bibliographic Retrieval Services. The initial file contained over 29,000 articles dating back to 1980.

Chemical Abstracts Service (CAS) was begun by ACS in 1907. Today, it is the society's largest staff division; it abstracts and indexes close to 500,000 papers, patents, books and other documents annually.

To create its database, CAS monitors some 12,000 sci-tech periodicals from over 150 countries in over 50 languages, patent documents issued by 26 nations and two international bodies, plus conference proceedings, dissertations, government reports and books from throughout the world. In 1982, CAS added 457,789 abstracts to its database for a total of 9.5 million abstracts. The database is said to require well over $30 million annually to generate and maintain.

The most comprehensive of CAS' publications is *Chemical Abstracts* (CA), which publishes some 8000 to 9000 abstracts every week. It is the largest abstracting journal serving a single scientific discipline, the oldest abstracting journal in continuous operation, and the only abstracting journal that still attempts to cover all information in its discipline.

CAS also publishes *Chemical Industry Notes* (CIN), a weekly compilation of abstracts, plus many other print services and reference works. In addition, it produces *CA Selects*, a current awareness service of 133 biweekly publications containing abstracts of literature in a specific subject. In 1981, CAS and BioSciences Information Service began the joint publication of *BIOSIS/CAS Selects*. This series of 23 biweekly publications contains abstracts from biological and chemical literature on topics spanning both disciplines.

Many of the print services published by CAS are also available in machine-readable format, and several are online, including CIN and CA SEARCH, the online version of CA.

In 1980, CAS began producing CAS ONLINE, enabling online searches of chemical substance information in the CAS Registry System. In late

1983 CAS ONLINE became a "subject" search system as well. The upgraded system may be accessed by subject index terms, keywords, bibliographic data and Registry Numbers in addition to structure searching. Answers can include CA abstracts and/or index entries. CAS itself markets CAS ONLINE; because it builds and maintains the chemical substance database used in CAS ONLINE, it feels it is best qualified to provide the most useful access.

Financials (in millions)

	1982	1983
Estimated Total Revenue[1]	$81.8	$82.7
Chemical Abstracts Service	60.0	60.0
Magazines and journals	19.9	20.8
Books	1.9	1.9

[1]Revenue from books, periodicals and database publishing. Excludes revenue from government contracts and other sources.

The American Institute of Physics
335 E. 45 St.
New York, NY 10017
(212) 661-9404

Representative Publications and Services
Physics Today
Chinese Physics
The Physics of Fluids
SPIN

The American Institute of Physics (AIP), founded in 1931, is a membership corporation with nine leading societies in the fields of physics and astronomy as members; these societies, in turn, have a total membership of over 62,000 persons. The purpose of the AIP is the "advancement and diffusion of the knowledge of physics and its application to human welfare," and it combines into one operating agency those functions, such as dues collection, subscription fulfillment and publishing, which can best be handled jointly by the societies.

The AIP publishes about 100,000 pages annually in 36 journals and one magazine, *Physics Today*. It also markets SPIN, an online database.

Physics Today, the official publication of the AIP, with a circulation of about 75,000, is sent automatically to every member of the nine member societies. The magazine strives to keep physicists abreast of all disciplines, and contains articles of general interest and of a cross-disciplinary nature. The main support of *Physics Today* is advertising revenue, which totals about $1.4 million annually.

The 36 journals published by the AIP include both AIP-owned publications and member society-owned publications; together these publish 80% to 90% of the results of U.S. physics research. A member society may choose to have its journal published elsewhere; if published by the AIP, however, the member society is only charged for the institute's services at cost. If the journal loses money, the society must still pay the AIP; if it shows a profit, the society receives it. Membership subscription practices within the individual societies vary; some send their journals automatically to every member, while others charge their members a special subscription rate. Nonmember subscriptions are solicited by direct mail, and most orders are from libraries. Most of the journals have a circulation of between 5000 and 11,000 copies and at least 40% of their circulation goes abroad.

Six of the journals, including *Medical Physics* and *The Journal of Vacuum Science and Technology,* carry advertising specific to the subject matter of the journal. The AIP has an in-house advertising division plus sales representatives on the West Coast and in Europe to handle advertising for these publications as well as for *Physics Today*. Some of the journals published by member societies also carry advertising.

Voluntary page charges are a large source of revenue for the AIP, totaling $2.1 milion in 1982. The AIP is probably the most important proponent of page charges today. All its journals have page charges ranging from $60 to $120 per page. Although they are voluntary, the institute will delay a paper's scheduled publication date by three months if they are not honored.

The AIP publishes 60% of Soviet physics research in its 19 publications that are translations of Soviet journals. In addition, in 1981 the AIP began publishing *Chinese Physics*, a quarterly that contains translations of the best articles from Chinese physics and astronomy journals.

In addition to its periodicals, the AIP also produces SPIN (Searchable Physics Information Notices), an online database. SPIN contains citations and abstracts to journals and conference proceedings published by the AIP and its member societies since 1975. Physics-related articles from other U.S. journals are also included. In mid-1983 the database contained over 193,000 citations and was increasing by about 2000 records each month.

Financials (in millions)

	1982
Revenue from magazine and journal publishing	$12.3

Engineering Information, Inc.
345 E. 47 St.
New York, NY 10017
(212) 705-7615

Representative Publications and Services
Engineering Index Monthly
Energy Abstracts
COMPENDEX

Engineering Information Inc. (Ei) is a not-for-profit organization recognized as the leading international publisher of multidiscipinary engineering bibliographic data.The company has been publishing since 1884, and is the largest engineering database publisher in the United States.

Ei's database incorporates over 2.5 million abstracts, representing a large variety of engineering subjects. Over 3500 journals and 2000 conference proceedings from 40 countries in 20 languages are used as primary sources, and about 9000 records are added to the database every month.

The organization's principal print products are *Engineering Index Monthly* and *Engineering Index Annual.* The *Monthly* contains an average of 9000 abstracts in each issue; the 1983 *Annual*, a cumulation of all records published in the preceding year's monthly issues, contains over 100,000 abstracts.

Among the company's other print products are *Energy Abstracts* and *Bioengineering Abstracts*, monthly collections of abstracts related to energy, engineering and bioengineering. Generally, these abstracts also appear in *Engineering Index Monthly.* In Fall 1983 Ei began the publication of *Engineering Information Technical Bulletins*, published both in print and on floppy disks for major personal computers. The bulletins, aimed at individual engineers, zero in on a topic of current interest in a particular engineering discipline. Topics so far include

Robotics, Nuclear Safety and Superalloys. Ei expects to publish four bulletins each quarter.

COMPENDEX (COMPuterized ENgineering inDEX), a machine-readable form of the Ei print database, is an online counterpart of the *Ei Monthly* and *Annual*. It contains over 1 million abstracts arranged and cross-referenced under more than 12,000 indexing terms. All data from 1969 to the present are online, and the database is growing by about 10,000 abstracts each month.

In 1982 Ei launched Ei Engineering Meetings (EIMET), an online database providing an index to the published proceedings of approximately 2000 domestic and international engineering and technical conferences, symposia, meetings and colloquia held each year. The database contains about 150,000 records; in 1984 about 100,000 records will be added.

In 1980, Ei established the Engineering Information Search Service (EISS), an information retailing service for engineering companies, consultants and colleges that lack trained information researchers. EISS will locate information on nearly any subject, obtain printed copies of any articles requested by the customer and even translate articles available only in the author's native language.

Ei's revenues were estimated at about $5 million in 1983; revenues were divided equally between print and online versions. About one-half of Ei's business is outside the United States.

Futura Publishing Co. Inc.
295 Main St.
Mount Kisco, NY 10549
(914) 666-3505

Imprint
Futura Press
Representative Publications
Pace
Modern Technics in Surgery

Futura Publishing Co., with estimated revenues of $2 million, is one of a group of relatively new publishers in the medical field that has chosen to publish clinical monographs in one or two specialty areas.

Futura specializes in surgery and cardiology and publishes about 25 monographs in these subject areas annually. Approximately 60% of its book sales are by direct mail, with the remainder generated from advertisements in specialty journals and exhibits at medical meetings.

Futura sells its books throughout the world and has representatives in Japan, Europe, Australia and South America.

In addition to its line of books, the company publishes *Modern Technics In Surgery*, a loose-leaf service. Six volumes of this projected 10-volume series on current operative procedures have been released thus far, and the company expects to publish two additional volumes in 1984. Each volume is devoted to one specialty, such as abdominal surgery or cardiac/thoracic surgery. Subscribers may purchase the initial volumes for $49.50 each, and individual volumes may be purchased for $59.50. A new installment is issued at least once a year for each volume; subscribers receive these updates automatically at an average cost of $35 each.

Futura also publishes four journals. *Pace*, a bimonthly journal on laboratory and clinical cardiac pacing and electrophysiology, has a circulation of about 5200. *Postgraduate Radiology, A Journal of Continuing Education* is published in cooperation with Louisiana State University Medical School; its 2500 subscribers receive Continuing Medical Education credits by completing questionnaires included in the articles.

Clinical Progress in Pacing and Electrophysiology, a bimonthly, was launched in 1983 and *Echocardiography*, a quarterly review of cardiovascular ultrasound, began publication in January 1984.

Harper & Row, Publishers, Inc.
10 E. 53 St.
New York, NY 10022
(212) 207-7000

J.B. Lippincott Company
East Washington Square
Phildelphia, PA 19105
(215) 574-4200

Imprints
  Harper & Row
  J.B. Lippincott
Representative Publications
  Journals:
    Annals of Surgery
    Cancer
    Spine
  Loose-Leaf Services:
    Clinical Dentistry
    Practice of Pediatrics

Harper & Row, Publishers, Inc., was established in 1962 as a result of the consolidation of Harper & Brothers, founded in 1817, and Row, Peterson & Company, founded in 1906. In 1978 the company acquired J.B. Lippincott Company; although Lippincott is maintained as a wholly owned subsidiary in the health professions publishing area, its operations have been substantially integrated with those of Harper & Row.

The company operates in three industry segments: educational texts, in which it publishes a broad range of elementary, high school and college textbooks; general books, in which it publishes reference books, adult trade books, children's books and books of religious interest; and professional publications, in which it publishes books, journals and other services in the fields of medicine, nursing and the social sciences. (In late 1982 the company established a new department, Electronic and Technical Publishing, which publishes computer software and books about computer software and hardware. The books and software are sold in each of the three industry segments.) In fiscal 1983 Harper & Row published over 1200 new books, films, tapes, texts, loose-leaf sets, electronic databases, and computer software and instructional systems, as well as over 40 journals and other periodicals.

Prior to early 1981, Lippincott's Health Professions Division was located in Philadelphia, while Harper's Medical Department's editorial offices were located in Hagerstown, Maryland. All book production, manufacturing and marketing took place in Philadelphia, however. In 1981, the editorial functions for both Lippincott and Harper titles were combined in Philadelphia under the J.B. Lippincott Co.

The company publishes about 90 medical and nursing titles annually. It believes there is an abundance of medical literature available and attempts to publish only the more substantial titles that it feels will make a contribution to the literature.

Harper publishes 37 journals and periodicals in the medical and allied health fields. Four of its journals—*Clinical Orthopaedics and Related Research, Clinical Obstetrics and Gynecology, Clinics in Dermatology* and *Problems in General Surgery*—are similar to W.B. Saunders' Clinics of North America. In 1983 it began publishing *Computers in Nursing*, a newsletter designed to meet the need for timely information on the current applications of computers in nursing.

Harper & Row is the major publisher of loose-leaf services in the medical field. Its 10 medical and dental services are multiauthored, multivolume reference sets offering comprehensive coverage of specific medical specialties, with continuous updating provided by means of an annual revision service.

In 1981 Harper & Row acquired the publishing assets of Facts &

Comparisons, Inc., a supplier of information to pharmacists. This subsidiary publishes *Facts and Comparisons*, a loose-leaf service containing data on over 10,000 drug products, including 3000 over-the-counter items; *Drug Interaction Facts,* a loose-leaf service based on a computerized database developed by Stanford University Medical Center that provides information on all drug interactions of clinical significance that have been well documented in man; and *Drug Newsletter*, a monthly letter summarizing information on new findings and recent developments in drug therapy.

In fiscal 1983 Harper & Row reported net operating revenues of $182,384,000, of which professional publishing accounted for $52,687,000, or 28.9%. Harper's publishing activities in the health professions totaled an estimated $50.6 million.

Hemisphere Publishing Corporation
79 Madison Ave.
New York, NY 10016
(212) 725-1999

Imprint
Hemisphere Publishing Corporation
Representative Publications
Numerical Heat Transfer
Pediatric Pathology
Heat Exchanger Design Handbook

Hemisphere Publishing Corp., which was established in 1973, is a publisher of scientific, technical and medical books and journals.

The company publishes 50 books a year, primarily in the fields of engineering and toxicology, and has about 300 titles on its backlist. Some of its titles are distributed outside the U.S. by McGraw-Hill and Springer-Verlag.

Hemisphere publishes 22 journals, including three nursing journals acquired from McGraw-Hill in 1980 and *Pediatric Pathology* and *Ultrastructural Pathology* in the field of pathology. Circulations of the 22 publications range from 400 to 3000 copies, and subscription rates range from $40 to $200 annually.

In 1981 Hemisphere began publishing the *Heat Exchanger Design Handbook,* a loose-leaf engineering handbook that is updated twice a year. It is the only service available to the public in the engineering field.

Hemisphere's revenues are between $2.5 and $3.0 million annually.

Institute of Electrical and Electronics Engineers, Inc.
345 E. 47 St.
New York, NY 10017
(212) 705-7900

Imprint
   IEEE Press
Representative Publications
   IEEE Spectrum
   Computer Magazine
   Journal of Oceanic Engineering

The Institute of Electrical and Electronics Engineers, Inc. (IEEE), the largest engineering society in the world, publishes 14 society-owned magazines and 45 journals, as well as books, conference proceedings and standards books.

IEEE tries to run its publishing operation in a manner similar to that of a commercial publisher. It does not knowingly take on too many projects destined to be unprofitable and unsuccessful; however, it may make more exceptions than a commercial publisher does. It also differs from a commercial publisher in that its 230,000 members provide it with a well-defined market for its publications.

The IEEE Press, which had 84 books in print in 1983, publishes reprint volumes containing selected articles drawn mostly, but not exclusively, from IEEE literature. It publishes several of these books a year, as well as conference proceedings and standards books. Recently it began an expansion program and is planning to publish 20 to 30 books annually, including original titles. Members receive a 20% to 40% discount from list price.

The organization publishes *IEEE Spectrum*—a monthly magazine sent to its entire membership—plus 13 other magazines, including *Micro Magazine, Control Systems Magazine* and *Computer Magazine*. It also publishes 45 journals, including *Power Apparatus and Systems* and *Consumer Electronics*.

An IEEE member is eligible to join one or more of its 35 member societies; about half of its members belong to two societies. Each society publishes at least one journal. Since the societies have memberships ranging from 1000 to over 40,000, with the average about 5000 to 10,000 members, there is a well-defined market identified for each journal. A society member may choose one or more periodicals in exchange for his membership dues and several others are available at reduced prices. The majority of nonmember subscribers to IEEE journals are libraries.

IEEE journals carry a minimal amount of advertising. *IEEE Spectrum*, on the other hand, carries product advertising, especially in the electronics area, instrumentation advertising, employment advertising and some institutional advertising. In 1982 it had estimated revenues of $4.8 million, of which $3.2 million was derived from advertising. In 1980 it introduced *IEEE Spectrum Select* (now known as the "Consumer Edition") a demographic edition that offers the advertiser 210,000 upscale readers in the United States and Canada and accepts advertising for selected consumer products and services, such as automobiles, cameras and travel.

IEEE's revenues are estimated to be in the area of $10 million, of which about 80% is accounted for by magazines and journals, 5% by books and 15% by its other publications.

Institute for Scientific Information
3501 Market St.
University City Science Center
Philadelphia, PA 19104
(215) 386-0100

Representative Publications and Services
Current Contents
Science Citation Index
Current Chemical Reactions
ISI/CompuMath
SCISEARCH

The Institute for Scientific Information (ISI), which was founded in 1960, is the only commercial publisher of scientific-technical (sci-tech) bibliographic information that deals with journal literature. It publishes several print services, of which *Current Contents, Science Citation Index* (SCI) and *Social Sciences Citation Index* (SSCI) are among the best known.

Current Contents, a weekly pocket-sized publication, contains tables of contents from about 1000 of the world's leading journals and from over 700 multiauthored books. Each issue is published in seven editions: among these are Clinical Practice; Engineering, Technology and Applied Sciences; and Physical, Chemical and Earth Sciences.

Science Citation Index, issued six times a year, is the world's only citation index to the complete range of sci-tech literature. Citation indexing, pioneered by ISI, identifies and groups together all newly published items that have referenced the same earlier work. Over 560,000 records are added annually and include all information contained in over 3300 scientific and technical journals.

The *Social Sciences Citation Index*, issued three times a year, provides the same type of indexing services for social sciences literature. Over 129,000 items from over 1400 leading social science journals are indexed; in addition, articles are selected from more than 3200 scientific and technical journals for their relevance to the social sciences.

ISI publishes several other indexes, including *Arts & Humanities Citation Index, Index to Scientific & Technical Proceedings* and *Index to Scientific Reviews* as well as several services in the chemical field. It also operates current awareness services and document retrieval service for articles reported, abstracted or indexed by ISI services. Until November 1981, ISI operated only two online services: SCISEARCH, and SOCIAL SCISEARCH, which are essentially the online versions of its two major hard-copy indexes.

In November 1981, ISI introduced three new online products: ISI/BIOMED™, ISI/ISTP&B™ (Index to Scientific & Technical Proceedings & Books) and ISI/CompuMath™. The ISI/BIOMED database covers over 1400 of the most important biomedical journals published throughout the world; ISI/ISTP&B is the only multidisciplinary online database of the proceedings and monographs in nearly every scientific and technical discipline; and ISI/CompuMath is a two-part package that provides print and online access to the literature of mathematics, statistics, computer science and operations research. Every item from over 380 key journals plus relevant articles selected from over 6500 other journals in the sciences, social sciences, arts and humanities is indexed.

Since 1981 ISI has introduced ISI/GeoSciTech, which covers the literature of geosciences/geotechnology, petroleum science, oceanography/marine technology, metallurgy/mining, mineralogy, meteorology/atmospheric science and related disciplines. The database covers 1978 to the present, indexing every significant item from 400 key geosciences journals plus relevant articles selected from an additional 6300 journals in the sciences, social sciences and arts and humanities.

In addition to the above activities, ISI operates a search service and markets Sci-Mate, microcomputer software designed specifically for menu-driven searching of online databases and for the management of textual information.

ISI's services are primarily used by libraries and individual researchers, with 2000 libraries worldwide plus some 30,000 individuals subscribing to its products. It is estimated that some 300,000 persons read one or more ISI publications each week.

In 1982 ISI revenues were nearly $24.5 million. About 50% of its sales were to customers outside the United States.

International Thomson Organisation Ltd.
c/o International Thomson Holdings Inc.
1633 Broadway
New York, NY 10019
(212) 956-6000

International Thomson Business Press Inc.
Two Radnor Corporate Center
P.O. Box 301
Radnor, PA 19087
(215) 687-9607

Medical Economics Co. Inc.
680 Kinderkamack Rd.
Oradell, NJ 07649
(201) 262-3030

Patient Care Communications, Inc.
16 Thorndal Circle
P.O. Box 1245
Darien, CT 06820
(203) 655-8951

Med Publishing, Inc.
50 Route #9
Morganville, NJ 07751
(201) 536-3600

Veterinary Medicine Publishing Co., Inc.
P.O. Box 13265
Edwardsville, KS 66111
(913) 422-5010

Van Nostrand Reinhold Co., Inc.
135 W. 50 St.
New York, NY 10020
(212) 265-8700

Representative Publications
Medical Economics
Physician's Desk Reference
Patient Care
Practical Cardiology

Veterinary Economics
Van Nostrand Scientific Encyclopedia

International Thomson Organisation Ltd. (ITOL) is a financial holding company for a group of companies whose principal activities are periodical, book and regional newspaper publishing; information services; the operation of travel companies; and participation in the exploration, development, and operation of North Sea and other oil and gas fields. International Thomson Holdings Inc. is the operating subsidiary responsible for interests in the United States.

In 1978 a major expansion program was launched to acquire and set up information, publishing, travel and natural resource businesses in the United States; since then, ITOL has invested $360 million in the acquisition of U.S. publishing companies. Its information activities in the United States include book, magazine, newsletter, database and looseleaf service publishing. These activities are carried out by eight corporations and their subsidiaries: Callaghan & Co. and Clark Boardman Co., Ltd., legal publishers; Warren Gorham & Lamont, Inc., publisher in the fields of taxation, banking, business law, real estate, accounting and medicine; Research Publications, Inc., a micropublisher; Thomas Nelson International, an educational publisher; Wadsworth, Inc., a college publisher; International Thomson Business Press Inc. (ITBP), publisher in the business and information services fields; and Van Nostrand Reinhold Co., Inc., a technical and scientific publisher. The company is considered one of the top five professional publishers in the United States.

ITBP was established in 1980 to acquire high-quality publications and to finance developmental projects in the business publishing and information services fields, concentrating on industries which are expected to grow significantly faster than the U.S. economy as a whole. The healthcare field was one of the areas it targeted for major growth, and it claims to be the leading healthcare publisher in the United States. It publishes magazines, newsletters and reference directories, has two professional book publishing divisions and is producing several online databases. It is composed of 11 companies, including Medical Economics Co., Inc., acquired in 1981 with the purchase of Litton Industries' publishing interests; Patient Care Communications, Inc., and Veterinary Medicine Publishing Co., Inc., both subsidiaries of Medical Economics Co., also acquired in 1981; and Med Publishing, Inc., purchased in 1980.

Medical Economics Co., Inc. began in 1923 with the publication of the magazine *Medical Economics*. In 1968 it was purchased by Litton Industries and became a division of the Litton Publishing Group. Currently, it is the world's major publisher of healthcare periodicals, publishing eight magazines; five annuals, including *Physicians' Desk Reference, Physicians' Desk Reference for Nonprescription Drugs* and *Drug Topics Red Book*; and specialized books.

Medical Economics is the company's largest magazine in terms of both advertising revenue and circulation. All magazines except *RN* are controlled publications.

The company's annuals are led by *Physicians' Desk Reference*, a complete directory of drug information, which is sent to over one million doctors and other health professionals annually. In 1980 the company introduced *Physicians' Desk Reference for Nonprescription Drugs*, the most comprehensive single source of over-the-counter drug information available. In April 1984 *Physicians' Desk Reference* became the company's first online database when it became part of PHYCOM, an online information retrieval service for physicians.

Medical Economics' book division emphasizes titles in fields served by the company's magazines, and the audience is limited to professionals in the healthcare field. The company also performs custom research for clients and has a division specializing in customized communications, including courses, seminars, booklets and single-advertiser journals.

Patient Care Communications, Inc., publishes *Patient Care*, the leading clinical magazine for physicians. The magazine, a controlled publication first published in 1967, is issued 21 times a year and contains clinical advice related to the problems the family physician faces in daily practice. Its major articles are based on the combined thinking of physicians from several specialties and usually include discussion of diagnosis, therapy, patient management and costs of care. The company also publishes the *Patient Care Flow Chart Manual*, an annual hardcover publication that is sold to physicians, medical schools and so on. The manual contains 295 flowcharts that are logical summaries of diagnostic, therapeutic and management techniques; these charts are a recycling of material that originally appeared in the magazine. It also produces special flowcharts on specialized topics (for example, the uses of a specific drug) that are marketed to pharmaceutical houses.

Veterinary Medicine Publishing Co., Inc., provides clinical and practice management information for veterinarians through the publication of two professional periodicals—*Veterinary Economics* and *Veterinary Medicine/Small Animal Clinician*, each the leading journal in its field.

Med Publishing, Inc., ITBP's first acquisition in the health field, publishes *Practical Cardiology* and *IM-Internal Medicine for the Specialist*, as well as several newsletters in the medical field, including *OB/GYN Literature News* and *Pulmonary Disease Literature News*.

Van Nostrand Reinhold Co., Inc. (VNR), also acquired in 1981 with the purchase of Litton Industries' publishing interests, is a leading technical and scientific publisher, concentrating on science, engineering and special interest titles and serving the needs of practitioners in architecture, engineering, computer science, gerontology, energy and business management. Together with John Wiley & Sons and McGraw-Hill, it is one of the three leading publishers of sci-tech encyclopedias. The company publishes 14 encyclopedias, including the two-volume, 3000-page *Van Nostrand Scientific Encyclopedia*, which claims to be America's most widely used scientific encyclopedia. In 1982 VNR formed the Scientific and Academic Editions division to publish specialized monographs, advanced texts, research and theoretical treatises, and symposia in physical, earth, environmental, life, and social and behavioral sciences. The company has also created a specialized journals division targeted to high-growth markets in selected scientific disciplines. This division publishes six journals, including *International Journal of Behavioral Geriatrics* and *Advances in Polymer Technology*, and a newsletter, *Data Processing Auditing Report*.

In spring 1984 ITOL stated that, henceforth, VNR would concentrate on engineering, architecture and design, food service and hospitality, business and management, and selected scientific disciplines for professional, institutional and higher education fields.

ITOL's 1982 sci-tech revenues are estimated at about $72 million, with about two-thirds derived from the publishing activities of Medical Economics Co. and about 15% from Van Nostrand Reinhold.

The Laux Company, Inc.
P.O. Box L
West Bare Hill Rd.
Harvard, MA 01451
(617) 456-8000

Representative Publications
  Newsletters:
    Infectious Disease Practice
    Collected Letters in Surgery
  Journals:
    Comprehensive Therapy
    Plasma Therapy

The Laux Company (formerly called Book Associates) publishes six newsletters, five periodicals and two loose-leaf services.

The five medical letters—*Collected Letters in Surgery, Collected Letters of the International Correspondence Society of Optometrists, Infectious Disease Practice, Money Management for Physicians* and *OB-GYN Collected Letters*—have prices ranging from $39 to $59.

Each of the three newsletters in the *Collected Letters...* group resembles an advisory service for a particular specialty. A physician will write seeking advice on the treatment of a problem patient; his or her letter is then sent to a panel of experts who attempt to answer the query. Both the letter and its reply are subsequently printed in the appropriate newsletter.

Money Management for Physicians and *Collected Letters of the International Correspondence Society of Optometrists* are sponsored publications, and in this respect they differ from most other newsletters. Several advertisers each purchase a portion of *Money Management*'s circulation. The editorial content remains the same throughout the issue, but each advertiser receives a four-page insert in his segment of the circulation. (*Collected Letters of the International Correspondence Society of Optometrists* is sponsored by a single advertiser that receives an advertising insert in the entire circulation of the issue.) The newsletter is then mailed to recipients selected by the advertiser and to some paid subscribers as well.

The company also publishes *The ERISA Newsletter*, a financial newsletter. In addition, The Laux Company sponsors seminars on subjects related to this newsletter.

Laux's five periodicals include *Comprehensive Therapy; Plasma Therapy,* acquired in 1980; and the *American Farrier's Journal*, which is intended for blacksmiths. In addition, the company publishes two controlled circulation medical magazines: *Medical Meetings Magazine*, with a circulation of 11,200 medical meeting planners, and *Hearing Journal*, with a circulation of some 13,000 hearing aid professionals and hearing specialists. The company also publishes the *Keogh Guidebook* and the *IRA Guidebook*, loose-leaf services with about 400 pages each.

In 1982 Laux's revenue was estimated at more than $2 million.

McGraw-Hill, Inc.
1221 Ave. of the Americas
New York, NY 10020
(212) 997-1221

Imprint
McGraw-Hill Book Co.

Representative Publications
The Physician and Sportsmedicine
Postgraduate Medicine
Washington Report on Health Legislation
Washington Report on Medicine and Health

McGraw-Hill is broken down into seven organizational units: McGraw-Hill Book Co. and McGraw-Hill International Book Co., McGraw-Hill Publications Co., McGraw-Hill Information Systems Co., Standard & Poor's Corporation; McGraw-Hill Broadcasting Co., Inc., and Data Resources, Inc.

The McGraw-Hill Book Co. publishes textbooks; trade books; educational and training materials; business books; and professional books in areas such as law, architecture, engineering, medicine and nursing. It also operates several book clubs and continuity series and produces microcomputer software programs and computer-assisted instructional programs using interactive video. The McGraw-Hill International Book Co. distributes many of the company's books and educational materials abroad, adapts and translates educational materials produced in the United States as well as by subsidiaries abroad, and publishes original works for specific markets. In 1982 books and education services accounted for 32.6% of total operating revenues and 26.2% of operating profit.

The Professional and Reference Book Division of the Book company publishes for the business and professional markets. Although it produces some books on purely scientific subjects, most of the approximately 150 scientific-technical (sci-tech) titles it publishes annually are in the engineering field. Together with John Wiley & Sons and Van Nostrand Reinhold, it is a leader in the sci-tech encyclopedia sector, with the *Encyclopedia of Science and Technology* its most important title. (In 1984 it published *Concise Encyclopedia of Science and Technology*, a one-volume edition of the 15-volume encyclopedia covering the 75 major topics and areas covered in the larger work.) Its major strength lies in its line of engineering handbooks and computer titles, however. In 1984 it expected to release several software titles in engineering fields.

Seven of McGraw-Hill's book clubs, including the Architects Book Club, Electronics and Control Engineers Book Club and the Engineers Book Society are in the sci-tech area. In addition, the Book Company also operates several continuity programs on topics such as solar heating and cooling and integrated circuit technology and applications.

In 1978 the Book Company established the Health Professions Division to publish medical and nursing books for students and professionals in both fields. The division publishes 15 to 20 medical books for students and practitioners annually. Most of its books are text-references that can be used in class by students and as references by practitioners. (In 1981 publication of nursing books was shifted to the College Division.) The division is the publisher of *Harrison's Principles of Internal Medicine,* a leading medical text that is a classic in its field.

McGraw-Hill's magazine, newsletter and newswire operations are carried out through McGraw-Hill Publications Co., which publishes business, professional and technical magazines, newsletters, newswires and other specialized information services for readers throughout the world.

The Publications Co., which accounted for 28.9% of total operating revenue and 24.0% of operating profit in 1982, publishes *The Physician and Sportsmedicine*, which has a circulation of about 92,000, and *Postgraduate Medicine*, which has a circulation of about 122,000. In 1984 *Postgraduate Medicine*, a monthly, announced plans to publish four extra issues featuring scholarly papers from leading medical clinics. Each "clinic issue" will include symposiums and editorial commentary about the evolving role of the featured clinic in the changing medical scene. In addition, the Publications Co. announced plans to launch four bimonthlies aimed at design engineers in communications, computers, industrial electronics and military/space in fall 1984. The company is also involved in Nikkei Medical, a Japanese joint venture, and licenses the rights to the editorial content of *Postgraduate Medicine* to Ediciones Lerner.

McGraw-Hill also publishes the Washington Health Letter group of five newsletters in the health field. These letters are concerned with regulatory and socioeconomic information and are addressed to anyone interested in knowing the effect of government policy on the health professions. They consider new medical developments only in terms of their effect on reimbursement, regulation and payment.

The editorial content of several of McGraw-Hill's magazines and newsletters is available on Mead Data Central's NEXIS system. In addition, the Book Co. has said it expects to offer the *Encyclopedia of Science and Technology* online sometime in the future, and in Spring 1984 the company announced it was developing a database that would make all its information products available online.

McGraw-Hill, with the vast information resources used to create its books, magazines, newsletters and other information services over the years, is ideally situated to realize the potential that the database publishing market offers. Its 1979 acquisition of Data Resources Inc., a leader in the field of economic information services, has provided it with expertise in integrating information, computer technology and customer support services. Combined with McGraw-Hill's own editorial and

Financials (In millions)

	1978	1979	1980	1981	1982	% Increase 1978-1982
Total Operating Revenue	761	880	1,000	1,110	1,194	56.9%
Total Operating Profit	142	166	189	204	228	60.6
Profit as percent of revenue						
Books and Education Services						
Operating revenue	305	335	355	378	389	27.5
Operating profit	46	49	49	50	60	30.4
Profit as percent of revenue						
Publications						
Operating revenue	232	269	295	332	345	48.7
Operating profit	44	52	57	62	55	25.0
Profit as percent of revenue						

marketing skills, this know-how should lead to a new generation of products and services in the TSM field as well as in many others.

McGraw-Hill's TSM revenues in 1982 are estimated at $62 million, with about 70% accounted for by books; 27%, by magazines; and 3%, by newsletters.

The Medical Letter
56 Harrison St.
New Rochelle, NY 10801
(914) 235-0500

Representative Publications
The Medical Letter

The Medical Letter, an independent nonprofit corporation similar to Consumer's Union, began publishing *The Medical Letter* in 1959; it is the company's only publication.

The *Letter* is a four-page biweekly that costs $24.50 a year; with a circulation of 165,000, it is the largest newsletter in the medical field and is read by physicians, medical students, pharmaceutical manufacturers, etc.

The publication evaluates new drugs and groups of drugs, and claims to be the only source of data on drugs that is unrelated to the pharmaceutical industry. Most of the information it publishes is available to all its readers; however, nonsubscribers do not have access to its evaluations or opinions on drug effectiveness.

The Medical Letter has four foreign-language editions which are printed in Spain, Japan, Switzerland (French) and Italy on a royalty basis. The French edition is also distributed in Belgium, France and Canada. The editorial content of these editions is identical to that of the U.S. edition, with the exception of some adaptations to account for different drug names.

The newsletter is also involved in a Continuing Medical Education program with the School of Medicine at Yale University, whereby subscribers may earn credits for reading the publication and successfully completing tests based on their knowledge of its contents.

Annual revenues of The Medical Letter are estimated at $4 million.

The C.V. Mosby Company
(Subsidiary of The Times Mirror Co.)
11830 Westline Industrial Dr.
St. Louis, MO 63141
(314) 872-8370

Imprint
The C.V. Mosby Company
Representative Journals
American Journal of Orthodontics
Heart and Lung—The Journal of Critical Care
American Journal of Obstetrics and Gynecology

The C.V. Mosby Company, founded in 1906, publishes textbooks, books for practitioners, and journals in the fields of medicine, nursing, dentistry and allied health. It claims to be the second largest health sciences publisher in the world and is the dominant publisher in nursing, dentistry and allied health. Mosby also has substantial strength in the market for college textbooks in the biological sciences, special education and physical education.

Mosby, which has about 2000 titles in print, published over 100 titles in 1982, including its *Medical and Nursing Dictionary*, which claims to be the most authoritative reference book available in the field, and ASSESS-TEST, a computer-scored simulation examination for professional nurses preparing for their board examinations. In 1982 it began publishing books on medical topics for the general reader, and in 1983 it established a software publishing division to develop computer software products for professionals and students in medicine, nursing, dentistry and allied health. Mosby also publishes videocassettes with accompanying texts for professionals in several specialized areas, including geriatric medicine and orthopaedics.

Mosby publishes 19 journals serving over 270,000 professionals in all phases of health care. Circulations range from 2300 for *Journal of Enterostomal Therapy* to 62,762 for *Heart & Lung—The Journal of Critical Care*. Seventeen of the journals are official society publications; three are in the field of dentistry and five in the field of nursing. All the journals are sold on a paid subscription basis.

Mosby's 1982 revenue is estimated at $46 million, with books accounting for $32 million and journals for the remaining $14 million.

New England Journal of Medicine
10 Shattuck St.
Boston, MA 02115
(617) 734-9800

Representative Publications
New England Journal of Medicine

The weekly *New England Journal of Medicine* (NEJM) published by the Massachusetts Medical Society, was established in 1812 as the *New England Journal of Medicine and Surgery* and is the oldest medical journal in the world. It has been called the "most authoritative source of medical information in the world."

NEJM follows the Ingelfinger Rule—named for its originator, former editor Franz Ingelfinger—in that it does not publish any studies that have been reported elsewhere; this applies even to newspaper articles based on interviews with the researchers in question.

In 1982, *NEJM* carried 4620 pages of advertising and had $9.9 million in advertising revenue. It appears to be the only major medical journal that publishes a regional edition; its New England edition is published once a month. The editorial content of the regional edition is identical to that of the regular edition; however, each issue contains advertising for local hospital suppliers, banks, real estate brokers, etc.

NEJM's circulation of 204,600 includes 11,200 copies that are automatically sent to members of the Massachusetts Medical Society. About 22% of its circulation is outside the United States, with about 7400 copies (representing 17% of foreign circulation of about 44,000) going to Canada.

NEJM has expanded its revenue base by publishing collections of reprints from series that appear in the journal. It has published several collections of its Drug Therapy columns, for example, and despite the fact that they were composed of "old" material, the first four collections sold 10,000 sets at $14 each in the first three years after publication.

The full text of *NEJM* is expected to be available online through BRS' BRS/COLLEAGUE information retrieval system for medical professionals during 1984.

Financials (in millions)

	1982
Estimated Publishing Revenue	$19.0

Plenum Publishing Corporation
233 Spring St.
New York, NY 10013
(212) 620-8000

Database division:
IFI/Plenum Data
302 Swann Ave.
Alexandria, VA 22301
(703) 683-1085

Imprints
Plenum Press
Consultants Bureau
IFI/Plenum Data
Representative Publications and Services
Handbook of Neurochemistry, Second Edition
International Journal of Thermophysics
Soviet Journal of Nondestructive Testing
IFI Comprehensive Data Base of Patents

Plenum Publishing Corporation publishes books, journals and databases through its Plenum Press Division, publisher of books and journals; the Consultants Bureau, publisher of English translations of Soviet books and journals; IFI/Plenum Data, producer of patent databases; and Da Capo Press, publisher of hardcover scholarly reprints of long out-of-print, virtually unobtainable books, primarily in the fields of music, jazz, dance, visual arts and the social sciences, as well as a line of academic/trade paperbacks in subject areas encompassing the arts, biography and history. Plenum also owns J.S. Canner & Co., a Boston-based company engaged in the purchase and sale of back-issue periodicals to libraries, colleges, universities and other users; Career Placement Registry, Inc., which has developed a database system of information concerning college graduates and experienced personnel who are seeking employment opportunities; and Plenum Video Programming, Inc., established for the purpose of entering into the business of marketing video programming materials to independent broadcasters and to public, cable and pay television networks.

The Plenum Press division publishes scientific, technical and medical books, including treatises, monographs and other advanced text-reference works, as well as meeting proceedings, works surveying the state of the art in various scientific fields, and specialized bibliographies and data compilations. In recent years a number of books treating scientific topics of interest to the general reader have also been published. During 1982 it published 301 new titles and had an active backlist of about 2850 titles. Plenum Press does not generally sell its publications to bookstores but instead markets them by direct mail and by advertising in scientific publications, including its own journals. In 1982 about 44% of the company's sales were derived from customers outside the United States.

Plenum published 157 journals in 1982, of which 62 were produced by English Language Journal Program of the Plenum Press Division. Under its Consultants Bureau imprint, Plenum publishes English translations of 95 Soviet journals, covering a broad scientific spectrum and, in 1982, published seven Russian books in English translation. This Russian Language Translation Program is carried out under the terms of a contract with VAAP, the Copyright Agency of the Russian government. The Consultants Bureau also has a contract with a learned society, whereby it provides English translations of 11 Soviet journals for publication by that society.

The company's IFI/Plenum Data division publishes and markets the *IFI Comprehensive Data Base of Patents*, a computerized index file containing references to all U.S. chemical and chemically related patents issued since January 1950. The file is sold to major industrial users and is also utilized by the division in its performance of patent searches for law firms and other customers. The division also produces several online databases for the searching of chemical, general, electrical and mechanical U.S. patents and publishes in book format the *Patent Intelligence and Technology Report,* the *Uniterm Index* and the *Assignee Index,* all of which are patent information publications.

Prentice-Hall, Inc.
Englewood Cliffs, NJ 07632
(201) 592-2000

Appleton-Century-Crofts Medical and Nursing Division
25 N. Van Zant St.
East Norwalk, CT 06855
(203) 838-4400

Imprints
Prentice-Hall, Inc.
Appleton-Century-Crofts
Representative Publications
Journal of Family Practice
Journal of the National Medical Association

The business of Prentice-Hall can be divided into four major product lines: textbooks and other educational materials for the college, elementary and secondary school markets; business and professional services; business and professional books; and trade books and other services.

Financials (in thousands)

	1982	1981	1980	1979	1978	% Increase 1978-1982
Net Sales and Other Operating Revenues	$30,055	$26,565	$24,461	$23,307	$20,824	44.3%
Subscriptions	14,363	12,288	10,567	9,540	8,584	67.3
Books	10,638	9,875	9,827	9,728	8,872	19.9
Database Products	1,999	1,770	1,403	1,162	912	119.2
Outside journals	1,795	1,832	1,703	1,932	1,755	2.3
Other	1,260	800	961	945	701	79.7
Net Income	5,184	3,728	3,510	3,247	2,663	94.7
Income as percent of sales	17.2%	14.0%	14.3%	13.9%	12.8%	

	1982
Estimated sales of sci-tech books (in millions)	$9.5

Prentice-Hall's scientific and technical publishing program is geared to professionals in electronics, engineering and computer science; most of its titles are sold by direct mail. It also operates three book clubs in the sci-tech field: the Electronics Book Service, the Builders and Contractors Book Society and the Behavioral Books Institute. In recent years the company has been actively trying to help general bookstores realize a profit on the sale of sci-tech books by means of an agency plan and a cooperative advertising program.

Prentice-Hall's Appleton-Century-Crofts Medical and Nursing Division publishes texts, reference works and journals for the medical and nursing fields. Its two controlled periodicals, *Journal of Family Practice* and *Journal of the National Medical Association*, have circulations of 75,118 and 25,521, respectively. In 1982 the division began publishing computer software for medical school students.

Also serving the health professions is the Robert J. Brady Co., a Prentice-Hall subsidiary located in Bowie, Maryland. This company is one of the leaders in the publication of textbooks for emergency medical technicians. It has also entered the personal computer book publishing market.

Financials (in millions)

	1982	1981	1980	% Change 1980-1982
Total Sales and Other Revenue	$409.7	$390.6	$353.4	+15.9%
Net income	36.3	33.8	30.8	+17.9
Income as percent of sales	8.9%	8.7%	8.7%	
Business and Professional Books				
Sales and other revenue	$53.0	$54.1	$47.8	-2.0
Income from operations	5.1	5.2	4.2	-1.9
Income as percent of sales	9.6%	9.6%	8.8%	

	1982
Estimated TSM Revenue	$36.8
Scientific and technical books	29.3
Medical books and journals	7.5

W.B. Saunders Company
(Unit of CBS Inc.)
West Washington Square
Philadelphia, PA 19105
(215) 574-4700

Imprints
W.B. Saunders Company

Representative Periodicals
Dental Clinics of North America
Otolaryngologic Clinics of North America
American Journal of Otolaryngology

The W.B. Saunders Company, which was acquired by CBS Inc. in 1968, is a part of the CBS Educational and Professional Publishing Division. This division is organized into five operating units: professional publishing, school publishing, college publishing, general book publishing and international publishing. The professional publishing unit is composed of Saunders and Praeger Publishers, a publisher of scholarly monographs and advanced college textbooks.

Saunders has been called the "world's leading health sciences publisher." It publishes books for students and practitioners in the fields of medicine, nursing, dentistry and allied health, as well as Clinics of North America, a series of hardbound periodicals, and, in 1983, six journals.

In spring 1980, Saunders became the first major U.S. professional publisher to enter the trade publishing field. The company, in cooperation with the American College of Physicians, began publishing high quality books on health-related topics for laymen.

Saunders also publishes 24 Clinics of North America, hardcover periodicals published three to six times a year which contain eight to 12 articles on a specific topic. The Clinics, which bear titles such as *Dental Clinics of North America* or *Otolaryngologic Clinics of North America*, are sold on a subscription basis and carry no advertising; subscriptions cost $22 to $64, and single issues can be purchased at premium rates.

In spring 1984 Saunders and BRS announced a joint venture aimed at developing information services for physicians and health care professionals based on Saunders' publications. BRS/Saunders Medical Knowledge Resources will have an exclusive license to distribute Saunders' publications electronically and will also distribute information produced by other medical publishers.

Saunders' revenue in 1982 is estimated at $54 million.

Springhouse Corp.
1111 Bethlehem Pike
Springhouse, PA 19477
(215) 646-8700

Imprints
Nursing Skillbook
Nursing Photobook
Nurse's Reference Library
Representative Publications
Nursing '84
Nurse's Guide to Drugs

Springhouse Corp. changed its name from Intermed Communications, Inc., in August 1983. It publishes *Nursing '84*, which claims to be the world's largest nursing magazine; *Nursing '84 Career Directory*, an annual publication that carries employment opportunity advertising as well as editorial material on nursing careers; and *Nursing Life*, a bimonthly magazine established in 1981 as a career-development magazine for practicing nurses.

Springhouse began with the publication of *Nursing '71* in November 1971 with an investment of less than $50,000. *Nursing '84*'s 1983 revenues are estimated at about $15 million, and the company attributes its growth to the fact that it is a quality product marketed with vigorous and aggressive selling. About 85% of *Nursing '84*'s subscribers are located in the United States and Canada; subscriptions account for about 60% of magazine revenue and advertising for the remaining 40%.

Springhouse also publishes about six books a year on nursing topics, which are marketed as continuity series to its magazine subscribers; it appears to be the only medical publisher that markets continuity series. Currently it markets three such series: the Nursing Skillbook series, the Nursing Photobook series, and the Nurse's Reference Library. The company tries to release a new title every two months. In addition to its continuity series, Springhouse also publishes *Nurse's Guide to Drugs*, an annual publication, also marketed by direct mail, which claims to be the most comprehensive drug reference ever published for nurses. The company also publishes non-nursing editions of several of its books under the title of "Professional Guide." These are sold by direct mail and in bookstores.

Springhouse Corp.'s revenues are estimated at about $32 million, equally divided between book and magazine publishing.

Technical Insights, Inc.
P.O. Box 1304
Fort Lee, NJ 07024
(201) 944-6204

Representative Publications
Newsletters:
  Biomass Digest
  Genetic Technology News
Reports:
  Molecular Electronics

Technical Insights publishes five newsletters: *Inside R&D, Biomass Digest, Industrial Robots International, Genetic Technology News* and *High-Tech Materials Alert*. These letters, which contain both scientific and policy information, are read by upper-level research managers who have broad responsibilities for new technology.

Inside R&D, a weekly, is aimed at research and development managers and deals with new technical developments and policies; it is priced at $312 a year. *Biomass Digest* is a newsletter concerned with the use of green plants to produce energy (gasohol or fire) and chemicals. It was launched in 1979 and costs $244 annually. *Industrial Robots International* was started in 1980 and costs $240 per year; *Genetic Technology News* was begun in 1981 and costs $248 per year; and *High-Tech Materials Alert,* begun in January 1984, costs $237.

The company also publishes a series of research reports on emerging technologies, covering topics such as heat storage and industrial robots. These reports, from 100 to 300 pages long, range in price from $85 to over $600. It is also preparing a directory, *Advanced Materials Research—A Guide to Experts and Opportunities*, for publication in late 1984.

In 1982 company revenues were estimated at about $1.6 million, divided equally between newsletters and reports.

John Wiley & Sons, Inc.
605 Third Ave.
New York, NY 10158
(212) 850-6000

Imprints
  Wiley
  Wiley-Interscience
  Interscience
  Wiley Medical
  Halsted Press
Representative Publications
  Journal of Clinical Ultrasound

Journal of Polymer Science
Head and Neck Surgery

John Wiley & Sons, Inc. is an independent publisher of educational, business and professional books; reference works; journals; and related learning materials. In recent years the company has become a major publisher of computer books and has entered into electronic publishing with computer software and databases offered online in the United States and Europe. In 1982 it acquired Wilson Learning Corp., a leading publisher of learning programs for industry. Wiley's publishing operations are divided into five sectors: the Educational Group, Professional Group, Medical Division, International Group and Wilson Learning Corp.

The Educational Group publishes textbooks at the college level in the areas of business, science, engineering and technology. It also publishes texts for courses covered in the occupational education market. The group has also introduced educational software packages in several subjects. Sales of educational materials accounted for 61.3% of Wiley revenue in fiscal 1983.

The Professional Group publishes books, handbooks, encyclopedias and research journals for scientists, engineers and business people. It includes Wiley-Interscience; Halsted Press; Ronald Press; Self-Teaching Guides; Wiley Law Publications, a subscription-based program; and The Wiley Press, a new imprint for microcomputer, small business and general interest trade paperbacks. The Professional Group has also entered the software and database publishing field and has published the *Kirk-Othmer Encyclopedia of Chemical Technology, Third Edition* online.

In the scientific and technical (sci-tech) publishing field, the company is predominant in the physics and chemistry markets and is a leader in computer books. Wiley, together with Van Nostrand Reinhold and McGraw-Hill, is one of the three major publishers of sci-tech encyclopedias and handbooks. It publishes four multivolume encyclopedias: The *Encyclopedia of Polymer Science and Technology,* the 26-volume *Encyclopedia of Chemical Technology* (ed. Kirk-Othmer), the *Encyclopedia of Statistical Sciences*, and the *Encyclopedia of Psychology*, published in 1984.

The Medical Division began in late 1973 as a natural adjunct to Wiley's publishing program. The company had a small nursing program and some basic science books on its list and regarded the medical field as a growth opportunity. In 1981 it acquired the medical publications of Houghton Mifflin. The division is a leader in the field of radiology and imaging, publishing the foremost periodicals in the area together with a complementary list of books. It publishes several series on nursing topics, such as the Critical Care Series and Wiley Red Books, which offer comprehensive, concise references for practicing nurses in all nursing specialties. Additionally, through a comprehensive library of medicine developed by the School of Medicine at the University of California, Los Angeles, Wiley offers internists a self-study program for continuing medical education credit.

Both the Professional Group and the Medical Division publish journals. The Professional Group publishes 78 titles, placing it sixth among commercial journal publishers, and the Medical Division publishes six periodicals. In spring 1984 Wiley acquired Scripta Technica, Inc., publisher of 17 technical journals, and also began the publication of its first magazine, *Professional Computing: The Authoritative Source for Hewlett-Packard PC Users*, a bimonthly.

Wiley is strong in the international sector. Sales of its International Group, which markets books and journals to professionals and students outside the United States, accounted for 24.6% of company revenue in fiscal 1983. Wiley is a leading supplier of books to China and has initiated a Japanese-language publishing program.

Wilson Learning Corp. produces management and sales training programs for business and industry in print, audiocassette, video and live formats. Wilson also designs special courses and provides consulting services for clients.

The Williams & Wilkins Company
(A division of Waverly Press, Inc.)
428 E. Preston St.
Baltimore, MD 21202
(301) 528-4000

Imprint
The Williams & Wilkins Company
Representative Journals
Pediatric Infectious Disease
Emergency Medicine Survey
Journal of Endodontics

The Williams & Wilkins Company (W&W) is the publishing arm of Waverly Press, which is both a printer and a publisher of books and journals. Publishing revenues accounted for 56% of total company revenues in 1982.

Books currently published and sold number more than 540 titles. In 1982, W&W issued 79 new books and new editions; of the more than 525,000 books it sold, 88% were in the medical field and 12% were in the

Financials[1] (in thousands)

	1983[2]	1982	1981	1980	1979	% Increase 1979-1983
Net Sales	$167,096	$137,201	$119,598	$103,290	$90,365	84.9%
Educational materials and programs	102,397	78,269	65,372	54,591	48,277	112.1
Professional and reference materials and services	53,018	49,832	46,212	41,196	35,187	50.7
Journals	11,681	9,100	8,014	7,503	6,901	69.3
Net Income	$9,584	$10,116	$7,452	$6,663	$5,786	65.6
Income as percent of sales	5.7%	7.4%	6.2%	6.5%	6.4%	

	1982
Estimated Revenues (in millions)	
Scientific and technical books	$38.3
Medical books	8.0

[1]Fiscal year ends April 30.
[2]Includes Wilson Learning Corp. acquired in May 1982.

allied health areas, including biosciences, speech and hearing, dentistry, pharmacy and veterinary medicine. Book sales accounted for 42% of publishing revenue in 1982.

In 1983 the company initiated a publishing program in the nursing field and expanded its publishing activities in the allied health field.

The company, believed to rank second in terms of sales of medical textbooks, has a commission sales force that calls on physicians in their offices or at hospitals. Sales are also promoted by means of space advertising, convention exhibits and direct mailings totaling 2.5 million pieces per year. Approximately 54% of W&W's U.S. book sales are made through wholesalers, and the remaining 46% are made direct to the consumer by the company; 27% of book sales were made outside the United States in 1982.

W&W first entered the journal publishing arena in 1909, and was publishing 48 journals in the medical field in 1984; 34 of these were society-sponsored journals, while the remaining 14 were company-owned.

The company attempts through its journal publishing program both to publish a product affordable to individual subscribers and to publish the best papers available. Most journal circulation is to individuals rather than libraries, with 27% of journal subscriptions going to foreign countries.

In 1982, a total of 219,453 paid subscriptions accounted for 72% of periodical sales. Revenues from advertising, which is sold by company salesmen, accounted for 17% of periodical sales; the remaining 11% of revenue was derived from the sale of reprints, back issues, microfilm editions and bound volumes. The company claims to be the leading commercial publisher of medical society journals and the fourth largest commercial publisher of U.S. medical journals in terms of subscription revenue.

Williams & Wilkins also publishes two Continuing Medical Education Programs, each of which is a 26-lesson home study course providing Category I Physician Recognition Award credit hours. In addition, the company is participating in two electronic publishing ventures. Its *Stedman's Medical Dictionary* (24th edition) has been converted into a medical speller for use with word processors in a floppy disc format by Dictronics, Inc.; W&W is the copyright holder on the spelling package. It is also a participant in Superindex, produced by Superindex Inc., an online database composed of title pages, content pages and indexes of professional reference books from over 20 publishers in science, engineering and medicine.

Financials (In thousands)

	1982	1981	1980	% Increase 1980-1982
Net Sales	$29,281	$26,851	$22,486	30.2%
Periodical sales	16,983	13,694	11,243	51.1
Book sales	12,298	13,157	11,243	9.4
Operating profit	3,265	3,347	2,498	30.7
Percent operating profit to net sales	11.2%	12.5%	11.1%	

Year Book Medical Publishers
(Subsidiary of The Times Mirror Co.)
35 East Wacker Dr.
Chicago, IL 60601
(312) 726-9733

Imprint
Year Book Medical Publishers
Representative Publications
Disease-A-Month
Current Problems in Diagnostic Radiology
Year Book of Pediatrics Newsletter

Year Book Medical Publishers, a subsidiary of The Times Mirror Co., is the smallest member of the Times Mirror professional book publishing group, which includes Matthew Bender & Co. and the C.V. Mosby Company. The company publishes yearbooks, medical reference books and textbooks, an "advances" series, journals and newsletters.

The company publishes 25 annually produced yearbooks, including *The Year Book of Critical Care Medicine*, first published in 1983. Each volume covers a different medical specialty and is a digest of literature from over 500 U.S. and foreign journals; the content is chosen by members of the specialty who may read as many as 20,000 articles in order to come up with the 200 to 400 articles included in each book. Each article is summarized in about 400 words with appropriate tables, figures and photos, and is accompanied by commentary by the editors and advisors. The yearbooks constitute one-third of the company's publishing program and account for 50% to 55% of sales.

Year Book also publishes five titles in its "advances" series, a series of annual volumes summarizing sophisticated recent medical progress in a specific field. Each volume is composed of original up-to-date summations of both the state of the art and the discernible future trends in the field written by leading authorities in the area.

The company also publishes seven pocket-sized periodicals with titles such as *Disease-A-Month, Current Problems in Diagnostic Radiology* and *Current Problems in Cancer.* Each issue is devoted exclusively to a single topic of major importance, which, in some cases, may be continued from one issue to the next. The articles do not represent original research; rather, they are summaries of research in specific specialties and its relationship to a practice. Each issue generally contains only one article, usually 60 to 80 pages in length. An editorial board decides on the topics to be covered each year and invites submission of individual articles; there is no peer review as such.

Year Book publishes *The Year Book of Pediatrics Newsletter*, a monthly letter reporting on developments in pediatrics, and *The Year Book of Urology Newsletter*, a monthly letter that consists of annotated abstracts of articles from the specialty literature, synopses of urologic conferences, summaries of recent meetings, announcements and so on.

In 1982 Year Book's revenue was estimated at $26 million.

Index

Abridged Index Medicus, 151
Abstracts of Entomology, 156
Abstracts on Health Effects of Environmental Pollutants, 156
Abstracts of Mycology, 156
Academic Press, 18, 20, 32, 33, 35, 47, 167, 173-174
Academic Press Series in Cognition and Perception, 32
Advances, 32
Advances in Agronomy, 32
Advances in Aquatic Microbiology, 32
advertising revenue, 2, 4, 7, 20-21, 78-83, 93-95, 105, 108-109
agency plans, 40-41
ALA, 59
Almanac, 44
AMA/NET, 155
American Association for the Advancement of Science (AAAS), 70, 86
American Chemical Society, 20, 22, 60-61, 70, 76, 85, 135, 152, 161, 167, 174-176
American College of Obstetricians and Gynecologists, 77
American College of Physicians, 100
American Health Consultants, Inc., 112, 115, 123
American Institute of Physics, 20, 70, 76, 86, 87, 89, 98, 99, 100, 176-178
American Journal of Nursing, 78
American Journal of Otolaryngology, 37
American Medical Association, 11, 20, 77, 79, 86, 89, 93, 100, 155

American Medical News, 86
American Medical Publishers Association, 18, 36
American Physical Society, 98
American Psychiatric Association, 43
American Psychiatric Press, 43
American Psychological Association, 160, 164
American Society for Surgery of the Hand, 90
American Trade Book Directory-1982, 40, 43
Annals of Internal Medicine, 73
Annual Authorizations Service, 103
Appleton-Century-Crofts, 36, 198
Architects Book Club, 46
Archives of Internal Medicine, 93
Archives of Pathology and Laboratory Medicine, 93
Aspen Systems Corp., 21, 101, 125
Assessing Your Patients, 48
Association of American Publishers (AAP), 4, 17, 18, 19, 25, 26, 40, 42, 44, 51, 52, 67, 102-103
professional and scholarly division, 4, 33
Associated Scientific Publishers, 154

BA Abstracts on Tape (BAT), 156
Back Pain Monitor, 115
Behavioral Books Institute, 46
Behavioral Sciences Book Club, 47
Benjamin, Curtis, 27
Bibliographic Retrieval Services (BRS), 23, 137, 150, 155, 156, 161, 164
Bioengineering Abstracts, 149
Biological Abstracts (BA), 155

Biological Abstracts/RRM (BA/ RRM), 155, 156
Biomass Digest, 114
Biomedical Foundations of Ophthalmology, 127
Bio-Medical Insight, 119
Biomedical Safety and Standards, 115, 123
Biomedical Technology, 115
Bio Research Today, 156
BioSciences Information Service (BIOSIS), 155-156, 163
BIOSIS/CAS Selects, 153, 156
BIOSIS Previews, 156, 158, 163
Bookazine, 43
The Book-of-the-Month Club, 46
Book-of-the-Month Club/Science, 46
Bringe, Paul J., 116
Builders and Contractors Book Society, 46
Business Publication Rates and Data, 71
Business Publishers, Inc., 111

CA Collective Index, 153
CA SEARCH, 132, 153, 158, 160, 162
CA Volume Indexes, 153
Cable Health Network, 80
Can You Prevent Cancer?, 43
Career Directory, 83
Caris, Theodore, 101, 102
CAS ONLINE, 136, 154, 157, 162
CAS Source Index (CASSI), 153
CAT, 36
CBS Educational and Professional Publishing Division, 37, 44, 201
Chemical Abstracts, 132, 153, 161, 162

Chemical Abstracts Service, 22, 132, 135, 136, 152-154, 156, 157, 158, 160, 161, 162, 163, 174
Chemical & Engineering News, 20, 70, 76, 85
Chemical Industry Notes (CIN), 153
Chemical Week, 70
CHEMLINE, 152
Chicago Herpetological Society, 111
Chicago Herpetological Society Newsletter, 111
Chinese Physics, 89
CLAIMS™, 132
Cliggot Publishing Co., 105
Clinical Lab Letter, 115
Clinical Medicine, 126, 127, 128
Clinical Neurology, 129
Clinical Ophthalmology, 129
Clinical Practice, 150
Clinics in North America, 37, 106
Collected Letters of the International Correspondence Society of Optometrists, 114
Collected Letters in Surgery, 114, 120, 123
COMPENDEX, 149
CompuMath Citation Index, 151
Conquer Your Phobia: A Guide Using Contextual Therapy, 44
Consultant, 105
Consultants Bureau, 89
Consumer Price Index, 18, 55
Contraceptive Technology Update, 115
Control Data Corp., 132, 136
CONTU (National Commission on New Technological Uses of Copyrighted Works), 102

Cooperative Advertising Plans, 42, 45
Copyright Act of 1976, 101-103, 163
Copyright Clearance Center, 102-103
Copyright Office, 101-103
Core Curriculum of Clinical Dermatology, 100
CPC Communications, 105
Current Concepts in Trauma Care, 105
Current Contents, 149-150
Current Problems in Pediatrics, 106

Database services, 7, 22-23, 49, 64, 83, 100, 101, 104, 123, 131-166, 169, 170
Dealing with Death and Dying, 48
Dental Clinics of North America, 106
Design & Test of Computers Magazine, 76
DIALOG Information Services, Inc., 23, 136-137, 155, 160, 162, 164
Discover, 70
DIMDI, 151
Disease-A-Month, 106
Diversion, 76, 78
Drug Interaction Facts, 125
Drug Research Reports-"The Blue Sheet," 111

Economic Disclosure, 105
ECRI, 123, 124
Ediciones Lerner, 84
Ei Engineering Meetings (EIMET), 149
Electronics and Control Engineers Book Club, 46

Electronics Book Club, 46
Electronics Book Service, 46
Elsevier North-Holland, 33, 36, 47, 57, 73, 154, 170
Emergency Care Research Institute, 123
EMPIRES, 155
Employee Health & Fitness, 115
Employment trends, 7-15, 27, 29
Encyclopedia of Computer Science, 63
Encyclopedia of Minerals, 63
Encyclopedia of Polymer Science and Technology, 62
Encyclopedia of Psychology, 62
The Encyclopedia of Science and Technology, 63
Encyclopedia of Statistical Sciences, 62
Energy Abstracts, 149
Energy & Minerals Resources, 111
Engineering Index, 137
Engineering Index Annual, 137, 149
Engineering Index Monthly, 137, 149
Engineering Information Inc. (Ei), 22, 135, 137, 149, 160, 178-179
Engineering News Record, 70
Engineering, Technology and Applied Sciences, 150
Engineers Book Society, 46
Excerpta Medica (EM), 154-155
Executive Fitness Newsletter, 111

Facts and Comparisons (Drug Information Compendium), 125
Facts & Comparisons, Inc., 125
F.W. Faxon Co., 70, 71
F-D-C Reports, Inc., 111
F-D-C Reports-"The Pink Sheet," 111

INDEX

Flow Equation for Composite Gases, 33
Folio, 76, 93
Franklin, Benjamin, 44
Freedom of Information Act, 164
W.H. Freeman and Co., 44
Futura Publishing Co., Inc., 22, 36, 179-180

Genetic Technology News, 114-115
Geriatrics, 83
Grune & Stratton, 174
GTE, 155
Guide to Biomedical Standards, 123
Gut Reaction: How to Handle Stress and Your Stomach, 43
Gynecology and Obstetrics, 126

Halstead Press, 203
Harcourt Brace Jovanovich, 33, 35, 83, 173
Harper & Row, 19, 22, 38, 85, 106, 125, 126, 127, 128, 129, 167, 180-182
Harrison's Principles of Internal Medicine, 26
The Health Hypochondriac, 43
Hearst Corp., 70
Heat Exchanger Design Handbook, 125
Hemisphere Publishing Corp., 125, 182
Holt, Reinhart and Winston, 44
Hospital Admitting Monthly, 115
Hospital Employee Health, 115
How You Can Help: A Guide for the Families of Patients in Mental Hospitals, 44
Human Sexual Response, 26, 39

IEEE Spectrum, 20, 70, 76, 97

IEEE Spectrum Select (Consumer Edition), 76
IFI/Plenum Data Co., 132, 197
IMS International Inc., 47
Index Medicus, 151, 152
Indiana University School of Library Science, 84
Industrial Robots International, 114-115
Infectious Disease Practice, 114, 119
Information Industry Association, 4, 102-103, 133
Information Service, 115
Inside R&D, 114
Institute for Scientific Information (ISI), 22, 135, 149-151, 157, 184-185
The Institute of Electrical and Electronics Engineers (IEEE), 20, 60, 61, 70, 76, 85-86, 97, 183-184
Intermed Communications, 38
Internal Revenue Service, 59, 99
International Bio-Medical Information Service, 110
International Copyright Convention, 52
International sales, 50-52, 83-84, 88-89, 121, 158
International Thomson Organisation, Ltd., 33, 35, 170, 186-189
Interscience, 203
ISI/CompuMath™, 150-151
ISI/BIOMED™, 150-151
ISI/GeoSciTech, 151
ISI/ISTP & B™, 150
ISI Search Network, 151

Journals, 2, 4, 19-21, 34, 35, 37, 38, 39, 61, 67-106
Journal of the American Academy of Dermatology, 100

Journal of the American Medical Association, 73, 77, 84, 85, 89, 93, 155
Journal of Clinical Engineering, 115
Journal of General Chemistry, 84
The Journal of Hand Surgery, 90

King Research Inc., 84, 103
Kivar, 57
Knowledge Industry Publications, Inc., 21, 110

The Laux Co., 112, 114, 119, 120, 123, 189-190
Leeson, Kenneth, 67, 72, 85
Lexan, 57
Library of Computer and Information Sciences, 46
Library of Human Behavior, Ltd., 46
Library of Science, 46
J.B. Lippincott Co., 38, 180
Little, Brown & Co., 19, 26, 39, 44, 57
Lockheed Corp., 23, 136, 137, 150, 156
Longman, 33
Long-Term Care, 113
Loose-leaf services, 2, 7, 21, 38, 125-129, 170

Machine Design, 20
Machlup, Fritz, 67, 72, 84-85
Macmillan, 46, 47
Frank Maga & Associates, 111
Magazines, 2, 7, 19-21, 67-106
   medical, 4, 39, 76-78
   sci-tech, 69-70, 75-76
Managing I.V. Therapy, 48
Massachusetts Medical Society, 86
Masson, 33

Masters and Johnson, 26, 39
Masters of Modern Science Series, 44
McGraw-Hill Book Co., 18, 19, 26, 27, 33, 34-35, 36, 39, 46, 47, 62-63, 80, 83, 190
McGraw-Hill, Inc., 190-194
McGraw-Hill's Medical Utilization Review, 113
McGraw-Hill Publications Co., 20, 21, 111, 112, 113-114, 119, 120, 191
Mead Data Central, 115, 123, 136
Medical Aspects of Human Sexuality, 77
Medical books, 4, 7, 17-19, 25-65
   book clubs, 47-48
   distributors, 39-52
   economics, 19, 26-29, 45-46, 52-60
   leading publishers, 19, 36-39
   library sales, 27, 45, 48-49
Medical Book Club of America, 47
Medical Devices, Diagnostics and Instrumentation-"The Gray Sheet," 111
Medical Economics, 20, 68, 76, 78
Medical Economics Co., 20, 83, 105, 170, 186
Medical Information Network, 100
Medical Knowledge Self-Assessment Program, 100
The Medical Letter, 21, 112, 113, 194
The Medical Letter, 21, 107, 111, 113, 119, 120, 123
Medical World News, 78, 79
MEDLARS, 136, 151-152, 160
MEDLINE, 152, 164
MED/MAIL, 100
Med Publishing, Inc., 186

Metals Week, 111
MINET, 155
Modern Medicine, 83
Modern Technics in Surgery, 22, 127
Money Management for Physicians, 114
C.V. Mosby Co., 19, 38, 43, 90, 95, 100, 167, 194-195
Most, Harry R., 25
Moynihan, Daniel, 60

National Commission on New Technological Uses of Copyrighted Works (CONTU), 102
National Enquiry into Scholarly Communications, 49
National Federation of Abstracting and Information Services, 133
National Institute of Health (NIH), 101, 102, 151
National Institute of Mental Health, 164
National Library of Medicine (NLM), 22, 23, 101, 102, 133, 135, 136, 137, 151-152, 154, 160, 163, 164
Nature Science Book Club, 46
Nautilus Press, Inc., 117, 118, 120
New England Journal of Medicine, 195-196
New England Journal of Medicine, 20, 73, 84, 86, 93, 94, 100, 119, 155, 195
Newsletter of Engineering Analysis Software, 111
The Newsletter Yearbook Directory, 21, 110, 111
Newsletters, 2, 7, 21, 38, 107-125, 170
NewsNet, 125

Nikkei Medical, 84
Nonprofit publishers, 60-61, 95-99
Nurses Book Society, 47 21
Nurses' Drug Alert, 120, 121
Nurse's Guide to Drugs, 39
Nurse's Reference Library, 48
Nursing '84, 39, 48, 78, 80, 83
Nursing '82, Nursing Management, 78
Nursing Photobook, 48
Nursing Skillbook, 48

OB-GYN Collected Letters, 114, 120, 123
Obstetrics and Gynecology, 77
Ocean Science News, 117
Oil and Gas Journal, 70
Otolaryngologic Clinics of North America, 106

Patient Care, 83
Patient Care Flow Chart Manual, 83
Patient Care Publications, 83, 186
Pergamon Press, 33, 73, 170
PHYCOM, 83
Physics Today, 20, 70, 76, 86
Physical, Chemical and Earth Sciences, 150
The Physical Review, 98
Physicians' Desk Reference, 83
Physicians' Desk Reference for Nonprescription Drugs, 83
Physicians' Drug Alert, 121
Physicians' Financial Letter, 105
Physicians' Journal Update, 80
Plant Disease: An Advanced Treatise, 32
Platt's Oilgram Price Report, 111
Plenum Publishing Corp., 18, 33, 35, 44, 84, 89, 196-198

POPLINE, 152
Postgraduate Medicine, 84
M.J. Powers & Co., 21, 112, 120, 121
Practical Cardiology, 79
Predicast, 108
Prentice-Hall, 18, 33, 35, 36, 46, 198-200
Prospective Payment Survival, 115
PsycINFO, 160, 164
Publishers Weekly, 25

Quest Publishing Co., 115, 123

Radiology Letter, 115
Random House, 33
Raven Press, 36, 57, 95
Reagan Administration, 164
RN, 78
Rodale Press, Inc., 111

W.B. Saunders & Co., 19, 37, 39, 43, 44, 106, 200-201
Saunders Paperbacks, 43
Saunders Press, 43
Science, 21, 70, 73, 86
Science Citation Index (SCI), 149, 150, 157
Science Digest, 70
Science and Government Report, 108
Scientific American, 22, 44, 127
Scientific American, 70
Scientific American Books, 44
Scientific American Medicine, 22, 127
Scisearch, 150
Sci-tech books, 4, 7, 18, 25-65
  book clubs, 46-47
  distributors, 39-52
  economics, 18, 26-29, 45-46, 52-60
  leading publishers, 18, 33-36

library sales, 27, 45, 48-49, 62
Sieber & McIntyre, 105
Social Sciences Citation Index (SSCI), 149, 150
Social Scisearch, 150
Solar Energy Intelligence Report, 111
SPIN, 100
Springer Verlag New York, 33, 170
Springhouse Corp., 19, 38, 48, 83, 201-202
Stability of Parallel Flows, 33
Standard Rate and Data, 70
Standard Rate and Data Service, 71
Stanford University School of Medicine, 127
System Development Corporation (SDC), 23, 137, 156, 164

TAB Books, 46
Technical Insights, Inc., 112, 114-115, 120, 202-203
Technology for Health Care, 123
Technology Update, 108
Technotec, 132
Theory of Optimum Aerodynamic Shapes: External Problems in the Aerodynamics of Supersonic, Hypersonic and Free Molecular Flows, 33
Thor Power Tool Co., 59
Thor Power Tool Co. v. the Commissioner of Internal Revenue, 59
Time Inc., 39, 70
Time, 70
The Times Mirror Co. Professional Publishing Group, 38, 208
TOXLINE, 152

TYMNET, 136

Ulrich's International Periodicals Directory 1982, 71
UNINET, 136
U.S. Court of Claims, 101
U.S. Department of Commerce, 50, 51
U.S. Department of Health and Human Services, 151
U.S. Department of Health, Education and Welfare, 11
U.S. Postal Service, 99
U.S. Supreme Court, 59, 101

Van Nostrand Reinhold, 18, 33, 35, 47, 49, 62-63, 170, 186
Van Nostrand Scientific Encyclopedia, 62, 63
Veterinary Medicine Publishing Co., Inc., 186

Washington Health Letter Group, 113-114
Washington Health Record, 113
Washington Report on Health Legislation, 113, 119
Washington Report on Medicine and Health, 113-114
Waverly Press, 39, 205
Weather and Climate Report, 117
John Wiley & Sons, 18, 33, 34, 36, 49, 62-63, 95, 203-205
The Williams & Wilkins Co., 19, 39, 87, 101, 102, 205-208
Williams & Wilkins v. U.S., 101
Women's Pharmacy: A Guide to Safe Drug Use, 43

Yale University School of Medicine, 113
The Yearbook of Pediatrics Newsletter, 38, 123
The Yearbook of Urology Newsletter, 38, 123
Year Book Medical Publishers, 19, 38, 106, 123, 208-209

Zoological Record, 156, 163
Zoological Society of London, 156

About the Author

Judith S. Duke is a former research analyst at Time Inc. and assistant to the director of market development at *Life* magazine. She is a graduate of Cornell University and specialized in marketing at the graduate business school at New York University. She is also the author of *Children's Books and Magazines: A Market Study, The Business Information Markets, 1979-1984* and *Religious Publishing and Communications,* published by Knowledge Industry Publications, Inc. She is listed in the 1982-1983 edition of *Who's Who in the World,* the 1983-84 editions of *Who's Who in the East* and *Who's Who in Finance and Industry* and in the 1985-1986 edition of *Who's Who of American Women.*

Other Titles from Knowledge Industry Publications...

After Divestiture: What the AT&T Settlement Means for Business and
   Residential Telephone Service
by Samuel A. Simon
LC 84-21301   ISBN 0-86729-110-9 $34.95

The Birth of Electronic Publishing
by Richard M. Neustadt, Esq.
LC 82-6614   ISBN 0-86729-030-7 $32.95

Protecting Privacy in Two-Way Electronic Services
by David H. Flaherty
LC 84-15492   ISBN 0-86729-107-9 $34.95

Who Owns the Media? 2nd Edition
by Benjamin M. Compaine, et al.
LC 82-13039   ISBN 0-86729-007-2 $45.00

The Knowledge Industry 200: America's Two Hundred Largest Media
   Companies, 1983
edited by Judith S. Duke
ISBN 0-86729-034-X $60.00

The Business of Consumer Magazines
by Benjamin M. Compaine
LC 82-180   ISBN 0-86729-020-X $32.95

Religious Publications and Communications
by Judith S. Duke
LC 80-17694   ISBN 0-914236-61-X $29.95

The Shrinking Library Dollar
by Dantia Quirk and Patricia Whitestone
LC 81-12319   ISBN 0-914236-74-1 $24.95

Electronic Marketing: Emerging TV and Computer Channels for
   Interactive Home Shopping
by Lawrence Strauss
LC 83-185   ISBN 0-86729-023-4 $34.95

Z 286 .T4 D84

JAN 15 '89
JUN 15 1992